Contents

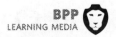

Contents

BPP
LEARNING MEDIA

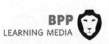

Contents

BPP
LEARNING MEDIA

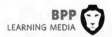

Contents

BPP
LEARNING MEDIA

About the Publisher

BPP Learning Media is dedicated to supporting aspiring professionals with top quality learning material. BPP Learning Media's commitment to success is shown by our record of quality, innovation and market leadership in paper-based and e-learning materials. BPP Learning Media's study materials are written by professionally-qualified specialists who know from personal experience the importance of top quality materials for success.

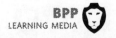

About the Contributors

Preface and Chapter 1
Graham Blackman, BSc (Hons)

Graham attained first class honours in Psychology at the University of Bath, which included a one-year internship at Harvard University. Since graduating he has held research positions at the MRC Institute of Hearing Research and the University of Nottingham. He is currently a final year student on the Graduate Entry MBChB course at the University of Birmingham. Graham is an enthusiastic teacher and has helped prospective students prepare for their Medical School applications since 2008.

Chapter 2
Sarah-Jane De Silva, BSc (Hons), RGN

Sarah-Jane graduated with a BSc (first class honours) in Nursing Studies from King's College, University of London. Following graduation, she held a position as a Staff Nurse at King's College Hospital before moving to work in specialist cardio-respiratory Intensive Care at the Royal Brompton Hospital and subsequently transferring to the general Intensive Care Unit at her local district general hospital. As a nurse, she has presented at National and International conferences. She is currently in the first year of the Graduate Entry Medicine course at the University of Leicester.

Chapter 3
James Rudge, BSc (Hons)

James graduated from the University of Sheffield with first class honours in Biomedical Science and is currently studying Medicine at the University of Birmingham on the graduate entry MBChB course. At Birmingham, James has previously held the position of graduate entry course representative, and continues to work closely with staff and graduate entrants.

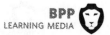

Chapter 4

Marco-Daniel Egawhary, BA (Hons)

After being awarded the Browne Scholarship in both his second and third years, Marco graduated from the Queen's College, Oxford, with a Double First in Biological Sciences. In his final year, he specialised in cell biology and infectious disease, and carried out research in HIV vaccination. Marco went directly into Graduate Entry Medicine at the University of Birmingham following his final year of study. In his spare time, Marco particularly enjoys teaching; having previously taught English and Medicine to pupils in Hong Kong and Cambridge (UK) respectively.

Chapter 5

Tim Spruell, BSc (Hons), MSc

Tim graduated from the University of St Andrews in 2007 with a first class honours degree in Human Biology. He went on to study for an MSc in Global Health Science at Oxford University prior to commencing the Graduate Entry Medicine course at the University of Birmingham. He is now a fourth year medical student, and is actively involved in a number of public health projects.

Tomás Donegan, BSc (Hons)

Tomás graduated in 2007 with a first class honours degree in Anatomy at the National University of Ireland Galway, where he has also worked as a demonstrator in the Anatomy department. He is currently a fourth year medical student on the Graduate Entry course at the University of Birmingham.

Chapter 6

Riaz Gulab, BSc (Hons), MSc

Riaz studied Biology and Toxicology at the University of Birmingham, and is currently pursuing a degree in Medicine also at Birmingham. Riaz has helped many potential medical students to achieve their ambitions of becoming a doctor. He holds a longstanding interest in working with young adults with learning disabilities.

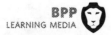

Chapter 7

Therapon Chrisostomou, BSc (Hons)

After obtaining a first class honours degree in Biochemistry at University College London, Therapon went on to join Birmingham University's Graduate Entry Medicine scheme as its youngest student. Currently in his final year, he has been invited to every yearly distinction viva along the way. Since starting his first degree, he has been keen to help guide and support students through their studies. This was established through his involvement with UCL's Peer Assisted Learning Scheme, which he continues to support.

Chapter 8

Anna Sherratt, BSc (Hons), PhD

Anna obtained a first class degree in Microbiology at Cardiff University. Her continued interest in this field led her to undertake a Medical Research Council funded PhD project on the structure and function of intracellular lipid bodies in Mycobacterium tuberculosis. Anna presented her work at both regional and national conferences and contributed findings for a published paper. She is currently in her fourth year of Graduate Entry Medicine at the University of Birmingham.

Chapter 9

Paul Mawer, BSc (Hons)

Paul graduated with a BSc in Medical Science from the University of Birmingham, and has now entered his final year of Medicine at the same university. Paul is extremely enthusiastic about Medicine and the exciting career that awaits him, but always has time for other extra-curricular activities within the Medical School such as rugby and the musical society. He wishes all potential medics and doctors that read this book all the best of luck and hopes that it will help them along their way.

Chapter 10

Dan Kim, BSc (Hons), MSc

Dan attained first class honours in Computational Biology at the University of Warwick where he was awarded the prize for Best

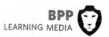

Overall Performance. He then went on to attain distinction award in his masters degree in Computational Molecular Biology, which included research at the Clatterbridge Cancer Research Trust where he was involved in Breast Cancer research. Since then, Dan has worked for the Health Protection Agency and is currently in his fourth year of the Graduate Entry Medicine course at the University of Birmingham.

Chapter 11

Michael Hurley, BSc (Hons), MRes, PhD

Michael Hurley gained a first class honours degree in Medical Biology from Brunel University. During his degree, he spent six months in the pathology department at University College Dublin identifying novel genes involved in melanoma. He also spent a further six months in the pathology department at Yale University looking into the early stages of colon cancer. Michael went on to pursue a Masters of Research (MRes) degree in Bioinformatics at Birkbeck College, London, followed by a PhD in Bioinformatics at the University of Cambridge. During the second year of his Graduate Entry Medicine degree programme at the University of Birmingham, Michael and his wife, Carolyn, had a baby girl named Ciara.

Chapter 12

Melanie Pearl, BSc (Hons), MBChB

Melanie attained a first class honours in Biomedical Science at the University of the West of England, which included a one-year placement at the Bristol Royal Infirmary. Since graduating, she has become a registered Biomedical Scientist in Haematology and completed the Graduate Entry MBChB course at the University of Birmingham. She is currently a Foundation Year 1 doctor at Weston General Hospital.

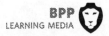

Co-editor

Ameesha Green, BA (Hons)

Ameesha graduated with a BA in English Literature and Philosophy from the University of Birmingham in 2007. Ameesha is a freelance editor, providing grammatical and structural proofreading and copy-editing to prospective writers. In her spare time, she also assists individuals with guidance on writing application forms and CVs.

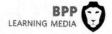

Acknowledgements

This book would not have been possible without the help of a great many people who have been instrumental to its development.

Thank you to Sabrina Chew and Ruth D'Rozario at BPP Learning Media who worked tirelessly to bring the book to fruition. Thank you also to Sarah Barnes for thoroughly proofreading the full manuscript.

Thank you to all the admission officers we contacted who have helped extensively in providing the details of the admissions processes and course structure at their respective medical schools.

Thank you to the Department for Business, Innovation and Skills for their help in providing the most up-to-date information on tuition fees.

Thanks to the following students who were so helpful in compiling the student reviews for each of the medical schools offering Graduate Entry Medicine: Sanjay Shroff, Dale Seddon, Lara Payne, Daniel Hughes, Laura Davis, Hannah Courtney, Thomas Reid , Ally Ellison, Barry Mullan, Matthew Harcus, Angelica Rohl, James Robinson, Peter Davies, Sarah Moorhouse, Thomas Lewis, Martine Mitchell, Mary Jarzebowski, Stewart Semple, Luke Turner, Jim Riches and John Williams.

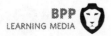

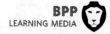

Foreword

This book is full of factual information and good advice to help you to decide, as a graduate, whether to apply to study Medicine and how to do it.

The book fills an important niche, since the entry requirements for graduate entry medical courses are much more diverse across different medical schools, compared to the requirements for those candidates applying at the school-leaver/A level stage.

I was pleased to be invited to write the foreword to this book because, as Medicine admissions tutor at Birmingham for the past 11 years (and having seen the inception of our own graduate entry course), I can vouch for the accuracy of the information it gives – and, of course, the book's lead editor, as one of our own students, has first-hand knowledge of our course.

Readers will find the organisation of the book follows a very logical progression. By the end, many decisions, such as whether to apply, which university, which course, and which admissions test will have been clarified. I thoroughly recommend it to all graduate prospective applicants for Medicine.

Chris Lote BSc PhD FHEA
Professor of Experimental Nephrology
University of Birmingham Medicine Admissions Tutor, 2000–2011

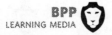

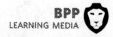

Preface

If you have picked up this book because you are considering studying Graduate Entry Medicine, congratulations, this could be the first step towards a life-changing career! Whether you are simply curious about the course, or are fully committed to the idea, this book covers all of the issues you may want to consider when deciding on whether to apply. In addition, the book provides detailed advice on the applications process; from completing your UCAS (Universities and Colleges Admissions Service) form to choosing which medical schools to apply to.

Purpose of the book

In case you are not already, competition to study aware Graduate Entry Medicine is tough! Medical schools are faced with the unenviable task of choosing applicants from a limited amount of information, yet their decisions can have a major impact on applicants' future careers. In addition, the added level of competition for places on Graduate Entry Medicine courses makes the selection process even more difficult.

As an applicant there are certain factors that you have no control over during the selection process, from the strength of the other applicants to the particular mood of an interviewer you encounter. It is therefore vital to prepare as fully as possible in the areas which you do have control over to maximise your chance of success. However, this takes time and energy and if you are like the majority of applicants, you will apply while either working or studying. Consequently, you are tasked with balancing your time between preparing your application and managing your other commitments. While a number of useful websites are available to help you with the process, the information is often disparate and sometimes inaccurate. Universities themselves offer information on their respective course, but collating information for the courses you are interested in can be time consuming.

In these circumstances, an accessible, yet comprehensive resource covering the key information can be extremely valuable which is exactly what this book attempts to achieve. Each chapter is dedicated to a different aspect of the application process, from

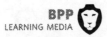

gaining work experience to succeeding at interview. In addition, major considerations for the prospective applicant, such as financing a second degree and returning to university are addressed in dedicated chapters.

It is important to note that this book is not designed to spoonfeed applicants through the process in terms of what to say, or do. Instead, it is written as a resource to assist you in submitting your strongest possible application.

How to read this book

Each chapter begins by outlining the content and concludes with a summary of the salient points. The book has been designed to be read either from cover to cover, or as individual chapters. A glossary at the back of the book provides a full explanation of some of potentially unfamiliar terms used in the book. As is the case with studying Medicine, conscientiousness is the watchword and it is important to refer to a broad range of materials during the application process. With this in mind, readers are directed to additional resources at the end of most chapters to further supplement their knowledge.

About the chapter contributors

This book has been written by graduates studying Medicine as a second degree, having successfully navigated their way through the rigorous application process. Contributors reflect the diversity of students on any graduate entry course, with some contributors commencing the course having just completed their first degree, while others have pursued a different career prior to deciding to study Medicine. However, a common trait in all of the contributors is a passion for Medicine and a desire to help other individuals succeed in their aspiration to become doctors. We hope you find this book a useful stepping stone towards a glittering career!

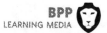

Chapter 1
Introduction

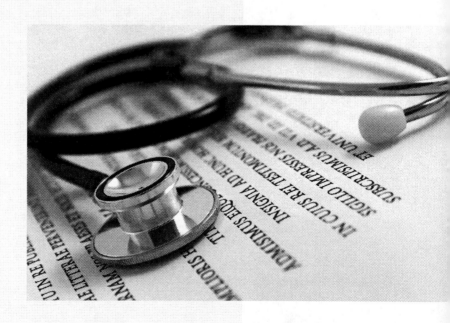

Introduction

Medicine is the science and practice of diagnosing, treating and preventing disease and has existed for thousands of years. Since those early days, Medicine has progressed at an astonishing rate and many millions have benefited from its advances from the development of effective pain relief to the introduction of vaccines. Medicine can be an extremely rewarding career and, combined with a huge range of opportunities to practice, research and teach Medicine, it is not surprising that it continues to be one of the most competitive professions to enter.

To become a doctor, the first rung on the ladder is to attain a medical degree which provides the necessary qualification to pursue a career in either Medicine or Surgery. There are various types of degree courses in Medicine and your eligibility to apply to these courses will depend on your particular academic background. This introductory chapter provides a short background to Graduate Entry Medicine and what graduate students bring to Medicine. The chapter then discusses some of the major considerations for applicants to Graduate Entry Medicine, as well as outlining the stages of the application process.

What is Graduate Entry Medicine?

Graduate Entry Medicine, also referred to as Fast-track, Accelerated or Professional Entry Medicine, is a relatively recent development in the UK. It offers graduates in the Sciences, Humanities and Arts the opportunity to complete a medical degree in four years, rather than the five or six years of a standard medical degree. The introduction of the course has created an opening for many individuals who would otherwise not consider studying Medicine as a graduate. This includes individuals who were unsuccessful in applying to Medicine as a school leaver, as well as those who only considered Medicine as a career option during, or after their first degree.

Although the course offers a fantastic way into Medicine for many individuals, there are a number of hurdles to be negotiated before you are able to call yourself a doctor. The condensed nature of the course means that it is, by definition, more challenging than a

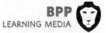

standard medical degree. Also, demand for places on the course is extremely high and as a consequence many strong applicants are turned away each year. However, for the well organised applicant, with the right academic and personal attributes – do not despair! Every year, many hundreds of applicants succeed in being awarded places on Graduate Entry Medicine courses and take their first step towards becoming a doctor. There are no guaranteed methods to securing a place on a Graduate Entry Medicine course, but undoubtedly, thorough preparation is vital to producing your strongest possible application.

Background to Graduate Entry Medicine

There is a long tradition of graduates returning to study Medicine as a second degree, with traditionally around 10 to 15% of Undergraduate Medicine courses consisting of graduates. For a long time this was the only route into the profession for graduates, however, this changed with the introduction of Graduate Entry Medicine in 2000. Two factors were particularly instrumental in the development of Graduate Entry Medicine in the UK. One was the predicated shortfall in the number of newly qualified doctors graduating from UK medical schools as the demand for doctors working in the National Health Service (NHS) increased. The other was the drive to increase the diversity of new doctors, as it had long been recognised that the intake of medical schools tended to be over represented by students from more affluent backgrounds (Department of Health, 1997).

From the small number of medical schools initially offering the course, there are now 16 Graduate Entry Medicine courses in the UK. All of the courses are based in England, with the exception of Swansea Medical School in Wales. Currently 11% of all medical students are enrolled on Graduate Entry Medicine courses, and while there is no indication that Undergraduate Medicine is to be phased out, the proportion of medical students on graduate entry courses is likely to expand.

What graduates bring to Medicine

Graduates differ from undergraduates studying Medicine in a number of important ways. Perhaps the most notable quality that graduates bring is additional life experience gained through

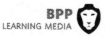

their previous degree, and in some cases previous careers. This generally equips graduates with a more realistic perception of what a career in Medicine entails and greater confidence that it is the right career for them. This can often manifest itself as graduate students appearing more focused and enthusiastic than their undergraduate counterparts.

As previously mentioned, graduate entry students tend to come from a more diverse background than their undergraduate colleagues. The age at which graduates start Medicine varies widely, with some starting in their early twenties soon after finishing their first degree, and others starting in their thirties (or even forties) having pursued a different career. Graduates' academic backgrounds also vary widely, with some medical schools accepting graduates with any prior degree. These factors combine to create an eclectic mix of individuals with a far greater range of life experiences than a typical undergraduate cohort.

Finally, graduates bring with them a specific knowledge base, or skill set that can be particularly helpful towards a Medical degree. For example, graduates in Biological Sciences will have a strong basis in physiology and pathology which acts as a foundation on which to add the clinical elements of Medicine. Applicants who have studied one of the allied medical specialties, such as Nursing and Physiotherapy, will have extensive clinical experience of different medical conditions. In a different, but equally valuable way, graduates with a background in the Humanities and Arts will have valuable skills in critical appraisal that are crucial in the current age of evidence based Medicine.

Considerations as a graduate

As a graduate, the decision to study Medicine can be more complex than as a school leaver. For example, you are more likely to be financially independent and therefore not have the support of your family for the duration of your degree. A significant proportion of applicants will have a partner or dependants which adds a further level of complexity. For those who have worked for several years, the practicalities of becoming a student again should not be discounted – for example, you may no longer be able to afford some of the luxuries you have become accustomed to.

Another unique consideration for graduates is deciding whether to apply to Graduate Entry Medicine or the standard five-year course. There are a number of factors to consider, such as the greater time commitment on the standard course and the greater intensity and competitiveness on the graduate entry course. Another key consideration is the financial outlay involved in undertaking the two courses, an issue that has become particularly relevant with tuition fee increases from 2012. Once this decision has been made, the applicant must then decide which medical schools to apply to. Each medical school has its own entry requirements and selection processes, making this decision crucial to ensure you maximise your chances of being accepted onto a course. Detailed information on each of the 16 graduate entry courses, including eligibility criteria, is available in Chapter 4.

Applying to Medicine

The application process for Medicine, either on the undergraduate or graduate entry course is both long and demanding compared to most degree courses. One reason for this is that medical school Admissions Officers act not only as gatekeepers to the medical school, but also to the medical profession in general. Therefore, a major role for medical schools during the admissions process is identifying those individuals considered to possess the right personal characteristics, as outlined in the General Medical Council's (GMC) publication *Tomorrow's Doctors* (2009).

So as a prospective medical student, what are the main stages involved in the application process? Firstly, having decided which degree course and which medical schools to apply to, you will need to submit an online application via UCAS. In addition, you are also likely to need to sit one, or more of the standardised entrance exams.

Assuming that your written application and entrance exam impress your chosen medical schools sufficiently, you will then be invited to take part in one or more interviews. Regardless of your written application, without a strong interview you are unlikely to receive an offer. Excellent communication skills are one of the most important qualities for a future doctor and the interview is still considered by many to be the most valid way to assess this

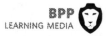

characteristic. Following this stage of the process, the medical school will decide whether or not to offer you a place on the course. If an offer is made, it is usually on the provision of certain conditions, such as gaining a particular degree classification if you have not yet graduated. If you do not receive an offer, or fail to meet the conditions of the offer, you will be faced with deciding whether or not to reapply the following year. There are exceptions to the above pathway, with some medical schools not taking into account entrance exam results, and others not requiring an interview; however, these courses are the minority.

A tough process certainly, but is it worth it? Absolutely. Despite the challenges faced when applying to medical school, once accepted you are on the first step to becoming a member of one of the most highly regarded professions. The degree still offers an almost guarantee of a job at the end and a structured career pathway to follow. In addition, the variety of jobs available to a qualified doctor is almost endless, meaning that there will almost certainly be a specialty that will suit your temperament and interests. An excellent starting point to get a flavour of the different specialties available with a medical degree is the NHS website on medical careers.

 Summary

- The last ten years has seen the emergence of Graduate Entry Medicine in the UK and there are now 16 Medical Schools offering the course.
- Competition is particularly high, with many more applicants than places; therefore careful preparation is crucial to success.
- Graduate entry students bring with them many valuable assets drawn from their previous degree and life experiences, making them particularly attractive to Medical Schools.
- As a graduate applicant, there are several additional considerations you may have, such as
  - Whether to apply to Graduate or Undergraduate Medicine
  - Whether you will be able to finance the course with an existing student debt.

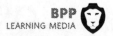

- The application process typically involves taking one or more entrance examinations along with the submission of a UCAS application.
- Once shortlisted, you will then proceed to interview which, if successful, will lead to an offer being made by the medical school.

 Useful resources

www.medschoolsonline.co.uk
www.gmc-uk.org/education
www.medicalcareers.nhs.uk
www.dh.gov.uk/health/category/publications
Department of Health, (1997) *Planning the medical workforce*, Medical Workforce Standing Advisory Committee, London

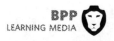

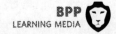

Chapter 2

Is Graduate Entry Medicine right for you?

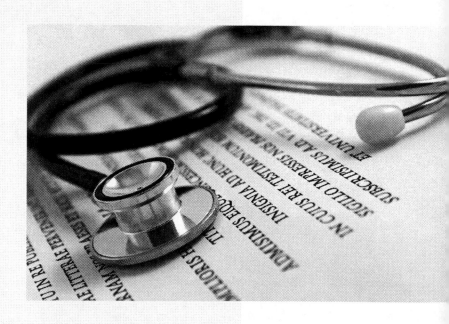

Is Graduate Entry Medicine right for you?

As a graduate wishing to study Medicine, one of the first decisions you will make is choosing which type of degree course to apply to. This decision can have a major influence on where you eventually study, how long for, and what form the teaching will take. This chapter provides an outline of the entry routes available to graduates applying to Medicine, highlighting the key features of the different courses to enable you to determine which would suit you best. The chapter also covers the practicalities of applying to medical school as a graduate, as well as common concerns encountered, such as the eligibility of your degree. The chapter concludes with a discussion on the relative strengths and drawbacks of Graduate Entry Medicine compared with Undergraduate Medicine.

Entry routes into Medicine

As a graduate, there are three entry routes to gaining a medical degree: the six-year foundation course, the standard five-year course and the four-year Graduate Entry Medicine course. Each is briefly described below.

Six-year foundation course

The six-year foundation course is open to applicants with, or without a degree. It is offered by a limited number of universities and typically includes a 'pre-med' year, which is aimed at individuals without the necessary science A levels to gain entry onto the four-, or five-year courses. Students study the basic Sciences (such as Chemistry and Biology) in the first year before joining students starting the five-year course. Generally, the academic entry criteria for the six-year course are equivalent to, or slightly below that of the five-year course. However, some courses have specific criteria regarding applicants' geographical location and social background. If you are considering applying to the six-year course you should contact the admissions offices of the medical schools you are interested in applying to directly, as only some will accept graduates.

Five-year undergraduate course

The five-year course is also open to applicants with, or without a degree, however, the majority of students on the course are school leavers, with A level qualifications predominantly in the Sciences. The number of graduate students on the five-year course varies markedly between universities, for example graduates form as many as 20% of students at the University of East Anglia Medical School. Conversely, at some medical schools, such as St George's, graduate students are ineligible to apply to the five-year course.

The five-year course also provides the opportunity to gain an additional degree by extending the course by a year, known as an intercalated degree. Studying for an intercalated degree enables students to undertake study in a particular field, usually in a subject related to Medicine, such as Anatomy or Medical Ethics. However, very few graduates pursue this option given that they already possess a Bachelors degree as a minimum. Some universities, such as Imperial College, only offer a six-year course whereby an intercalated degree is a compulsory component of the undergraduate course.

Regarding academic entrance criteria, most universities require three to four good A level passes (typically grade A), with Chemistry as an essential subject. Although having a degree is not essential for entry onto the five-year course, most universities state that where a degree is offered, at least a 2:1 classification should have been predicted or achieved. If you have obtained a good degree classification and possess a Chemistry A level, but your A level grades do not meet the course requirements, it is worthwhile contacting the admissions office directly to discuss your individual situation, as some universities will accept slightly lower A level results if these are compensated by a good degree classification.

Four-year graduate entry course

Finally, the four-year Graduate Entry Medicine course, which is the focus for the remainder of the chapter, is the most intensive of the three options given the accelerated nature of the programme. At most courses, students cover the first two years of the five-year syllabus in one year, before entering the third year of the five-year course. Some graduate entry courses allow students to intercalate

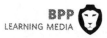

during the course, to gain a Bachelors or a Masters degree, however this option is rarely taken up by graduates.

What is the difference between Graduate Entry Medicine and Undergraduate Medicine?

Graduate Entry Medicine has existed in the UK since 2000 and is the most recently introduced route into Medicine. The concept is partly based on established models of studying Medicine as a graduate from other countries (such as the United States, where all medical students have a prior degree). The number of universities offering Graduate Entry Medicine and the number of places available on each course has increased substantially over the last decade, however, the total number of students on graduate entry courses remains relatively small compared to those studying on the undergraduate course.

In terms of pre-clinical content, graduate entry and undergraduate students cover the same core syllabus, ensuring that both courses comply with the recommendations set by the GMC. However, as stated earlier, Graduate Entry Medicine courses generally cover the pre-clinical syllabus in a shorter period. There are various rationales behind the ability of the course to reduce the length of the pre-clinical part of the medical degree without it being detrimental to students' learning. One is that graduates have already acquired the study skills from their first degree to learn the pre-clinical component of the course more quickly. Also, the majority of graduate entry courses require students to have taken degrees with some component of Biology, thus negating the need to cover certain topics during the course. In addition, graduate entry students typically complete fewer special study modules (where students pursue a topic of interest) during the first year than their undergraduate counterparts, allowing a greater proportion of their time to be dedicated towards the core curriculum.

In terms of clinical content, the GMC requires that the majority of the final two and a half years of a medical degree be clinically based, regardless of whether it is a graduate entry or a five-year course. In practice, the majority of undergraduate and graduate entry courses are clinically based for the final three years of the course. At medical schools that run both courses, the majority integrate the graduate course with the undergraduate course for the clinical years.

This integration with the five-year course has the advantage of enabling graduate entry students to benefit from being part of a well established programme. Also, the union of the two groups can be stimulating as knowledge and experiences are shared across the two groups. However, some graduate students may find it difficult to work alongside students on the five-year course, some of whom may be considerably younger than themselves. Furthermore, the expansion of the year group, from a small (and often close) cohort, to one much larger may seem a little disorientating at first. In light of this, it is worthwhile considering when selecting the medical schools to apply to, whether you wish to study with standard course students during the clinical phase, or whether you would prefer a graduate only cohort.

Another difference between the two courses is the teaching style, with graduate entry courses generally incorporating a greater proportion of self-directed learning compared to the five-year course. The rationale for this is that Graduate Entry Medicine lends itself particularly well to these learning approaches, because students have already developed effective learning practices. In addition, given that most graduates will have acquired knowledge of certain areas of the syllabus during the course of their previous degree, they are in a better position to know in which areas they need to invest their time.

Typically, the number of students admitted onto the Graduate Entry Medicine course at each medical school is much lower than on the standard five-year course. In the UK, the average cohort on the graduate entry course is 52 students, compared with 234 students on the standard five-year course. In addition, the characteristics of the two student groups differ, as the Graduate Entry Medicine course typically has a more diverse student intake than the five-year course, with students coming from a range of educational and professional backgrounds.

While the majority of students on the undergraduate course will not be educated beyond A level standard, all students on the Graduate Entry Medicine course will be educated to at least degree

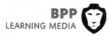

level, which impacts on the course entrance criteria. Although requirements vary between universities, typically Admissions Officers for the graduate entry course will be less concerned with A level achievements than the standard course. However, some Graduate Entry Medicine courses do stipulate that certain subjects be studied to A level standard (such as Chemistry) and most medical schools require applicants to hold, or be predicted a minimum of an upper second class honours degree.

Finally, another major difference between the four- and five-year course is the level of funding available. Home students starting Graduate Entry Medicine in 2012 are eligible for an NHS bursary towards tuition fees during years two to four of the course, whereas students on the undergraduate course are only eligible for a bursary in the final year. Similarly, home graduate entry students are eligible for an income assessed NHS bursary towards maintenance from year two, whereas students on the Undergraduate course are only eligible for a maintenance bursary in the final year of study. Therefore, the additional funding available on the four-year course provides a major incentive for many applicants, over the five-year course.

Can I study Graduate Entry Medicine if I have an Arts degree?

It is certainly possible to study Graduate Entry Medicine with an Arts degree. Currently half of all the medical schools offering Graduate Entry Medicine consider applications from individuals without Science degrees. However, it is important to note that of this group, the majority require one or more Sciences to have been studied at A level. Consequently, if you have an Arts degree and no Science A level qualifications, the number of universities that you can apply to is severely limited. It is also worth noting that some universities distinguish between life Science degrees, such as Biomedical Science, and non-life Science degrees, such as Nursing. Therefore, even if you possess a Science degree, you must check that your particular degree is accepted at the medical schools you intend to apply to. For the specific entry requirements of each medical school, please refer to Chapter 4.

What if I obtained a 2:2 degree?

Having a lower second class degree classification does not exclude you from applying to the Graduate Entry Medicine course, although it does limit the number of institutions that you can apply to. Currently, only St George's Medical School and Nottingham Medical School consider applications from those with a 2:2 classification. King's College London and the University of London will consider applications from individuals with a 2:2 classification, provided a postgraduate degree, such as an MSc or PhD has been achieved. Therefore, if you intend to apply to Graduate Entry Medicine with a 2:2 degree, it may be worthwhile considering undertaking a higher degree.

Is there an upper age limit for the Graduate Entry Medicine course?

There are several advantages to starting medical school as a mature student, such as the greater life experience that you are able to apply to a clinical environment and it could be argued that those universities running graduate entry courses particularly value these additional skills offered by mature students. Furthermore, the GMC states that the selection of medical students should comply with current equal opportunity legislation; therefore institutions are prohibited from discriminating against candidates solely on the basis of age. However, some medical schools advise applicants over the age of 35 years to seriously consider the implications of changing to a medical career. Other universities have stated that they expect students to be able to offer 25 years of service after graduation to the NHS. It is also worth considering that after completing medical school, you will have another five to ten years of training (or possibly more) before you be able to practise as a consultant or GP. Consequently, if you are 35, or over it is worth spending some time researching medical schools that you are interested in applying to on their particular outlook toward older students.

I have children – can I still study Graduate Entry Medicine?

It is certainly possible to study Graduate Entry Medicine if you have children and many parents have done so successfully. However,

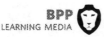

having children does raise additional issues, such as the amount of support you have at your disposal, which you should consider before commencing the course. If you require childcare, you may wish to contact the medical school you are applying to, as some universities offer nursery facilities. Although financial support for childcare is available for full time students through the Department of Education and Skills, you should nevertheless carefully consider the financial implications of paying for childcare while studying for a medical degree.

During the clinical placements that form a part of the medical degree, you will be designated to various hospital or GP practices which may be a long distance from your home. Although some universities consider personal circumstances when placing students, you should contact your chosen university directly to establish whether this is the case. A further challenge to parents on the Graduate Entry Medicine course is that at certain times of your training you will be expected to shadow doctors during their on-call rotas, which are typically outside normal working hours. Although challenging, by having flexible childcare and planning early you will be able to avoid missing out on these valuable learning opportunities.

How competitive is Graduate Entry Medicine?

Admissions Officers continue to see an increase in the number of applicants to medical school. Competition for Graduate Entry Medicine places is generally greater than for the five-year course, with statistics suggesting that applicants have on average a 38% chance of gaining a place on a five-year course, compared with 16% on the graduate entry course. This high level of competition for places on the graduate entry course can be explained by a number of factors.

One reason is that Graduate Entry Medicine attracts a broad spectrum of applicants, ranging from those wishing to change career, to those just finishing their first degree. Another reason is that there are fewer places on the graduate course compared to the five-year course, further increasing the ratio of applicants to places. In light of this stiff competition, many applicants choose to apply to both the graduate entry and standard courses in order to increase their chances of gaining a place at medical school.

As with any course, the competition for places varies between universities. Some courses, such as King's College, have in excess of fifty applicants per place making entry onto the course extremely competitive. However, the number of applicants per place is not the only indicator of how difficult it is to gain a place on a particular course, as it is also important to consider the average strength of candidates. For example, the University of Birmingham report generally only admitting those applicants with a first class honours degree.

A common concern for applicants to Graduate Entry Medicine is whether they will be able to pass the medical school entrance exam and proceed to interview. Presently the two examinations used by medical schools are the UK Clinical Aptitude Test (UKCAT) and the Graduate Australian Medicine Schools Admissions Test (GAMSAT). Universities vary widely in how the results are used to select applicants for interview. Some courses, such as King's College London, only offer interviews to applicants who score above a certain percentile of all the applicants. However, most courses consider the results of admissions tests alongside other sources of information, such as the UCAS statement and academic qualifications. It is therefore important to know, prior to applying to a course, how the results of an admission test will be used. It is also worthwhile to note that if you found a particular entrance exam difficult, it is likely that your peers also found it challenging and your score will reflect this. Furthermore, as some applicants will purposefully avoid applying to courses requiring a particular entrance exam, this may actually have the effect of increasing your chances of gaining entry to these medical schools by reducing the competition for places.

Statistically, securing an interview is the most competitive stage of the application process. The number of applicants interviewed per place varies between medical schools, for example on average Keele University interviews one applicant per place, whereas King's College interviews approximately seven applicants per place. However, if you compare this to the ratio of applicants to interviewees it is apparent that the likelihood of securing a place, once you have been invited to interview, increases greatly.

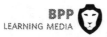

Should I apply to Graduate Entry Medicine or the five-year course?

Embarking on a medical career is a substantial commitment and one which you will no doubt contemplate seriously before deciding to apply. Once the decision to study Medicine has been made, it is advisable to deliberate over which of the three types of medical degree is the most appropriate for you. This is a crucial decision as it will not only affect your chances of gaining a place, but also how much you will enjoy studying Medicine.

There are a number of factors to consider when making this decision, such as the pace of the course. This is particularly relevant when comparing the graduate entry course with the standard five-year course, as the first year to 18 months of the Graduate Entry Medicine course tends to be very intensive compared to the standard course. Furthermore, as the graduate entry course typically includes a greater degree of self-directed study than the five-year programme, you should decide whether your learning style is suited towards independent study, or whether you prefer greater direction in your learning.

You should also think about how important it is for you to be able to pursue Student-Selected Components (SSCs) during the pre-clinical period, as this is generally reduced on the graduate entry course. However, if you are prepared to forego this option then the graduate entry course may be more suitable. Ultimately, when considering the advantages and disadvantages of each course, remember that at most medical schools graduate entry students integrate with their five-year counterparts after the first year to 18 months, after which there will be little, if any discernable difference between the courses.

Who make better doctors – undergraduate or graduate entry students?

The question of whether the graduate entry or the standard five-year course produces better doctors remains a controversial one. On the one hand, graduate entry doctors may command greater respect than their peers due to the greater life experience that they bring to their role as doctors. On the other hand, some may be cynical of graduate entry doctors as they perceive a career change

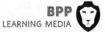

to indicate a lack of commitment and perseverance. However, it is generally acknowledged that Graduate Entry Medicine doctors often integrate into their medical career more easily than undergraduate doctors and become settled in their clinical roles sooner. It has also been suggested that in their early career, Graduate Entry Medicine doctors are more adept at appreciating the wider clinical picture than their undergraduate counterparts.

Research in this area has focused on comparing the examination performance of graduate entry and non-graduate entry medical students. A study of medical students at Leicester and Warwick Medical Schools by Carter and Peile in 2007 found that graduate entry students performed similarly to their undergraduate counterparts during the pre-clinical phase of the course (focused on the scientific basis of Medicine), however those with a background in healthcare were more likely to achieve higher marks in clinically based assessments during the latter years of the course. A retrospective study by Calvert and colleagues in 2009 at the University of Birmingham found that examination performance of Graduate Entry Medicine students was significantly higher than students on the five-year course. In contrast, a study of medical students at the University of Nottingham by Manning and Garrud also in 2009 found that academic success was comparable between students on both courses. In terms of clinical skills and preparation for life as a junior doctor, a study by Dean and colleagues of medical students in Australia in 2003 found that graduates on the four-year course were as equally prepared as their colleagues from the traditional course. Moreover, they considered themselves better prepared than their five-year counterparts in certain areas, such as interpersonal skills, confidence, and self-directed learning.

The Graduate Entry Medicine course is intensive and demands a high level of commitment, which itself generally ensures that those graduating from the course are highly motivated individuals. Furthermore, the graduate course generally includes a greater amount of self-directed study which serves graduates well for their future career. However, this generalisation does not hold true for all courses and some undergraduate courses also incorporate a large degree of self-directed study. Consequently, while it is not possible to determine whether Graduate Entry Medicine makes better doctors, students on the course perform at least as well as

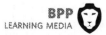

their counterparts on the undergraduate course and, furthermore, tend to excel in certain aspects of their medical training.

 Summary

- There are three entry routes available for graduates wishing to study Medicine:
  - The foundation six-year course
  - The standard five-year course
  - The four-year graduate entry course
- Several factors are important when considering which course to apply to which require careful consideration:
  - Courses vary markedly in terms of qualifications required and at what grade.
  - While all the courses are demanding, the graduate entry course at most medical schools is particularly intense during the first 12 to 18 months.
  - Being a parent, or an older applicant does not exclude you from studying Graduate Entry Medicine; however, some universities favour those under 35 years of age.
  - There are major differences in funding availability between the two courses with an NHS bursary towards tuition fees and maintenance available from year two on the graduate entry course, compared with year five only on the undergraduate course.
  - You should take time to consider the teaching style used and whether this corresponds with your preferred style of learning.

References

Calvert et al. Exam performance of graduate entry medical students compared to mainstream. *JRSM* 2009; 102: 425–430.

Carter Y H, Peile E. Graduate entry medicine: high aspirations at birth. *Clin Med*. 7: 2007; 143–147.

Dean S J et al. Preparedness for hospital practice amongst graduates of a problem-based, graduate-entry medical programme. *Med J Aust.* 2003; 178: 163–167.

Manning G, Garrud P. Comparative attainment of the five year undergraduate and four year graduate entry medical students moving into foundation training. *BMC Med Edu.* 2009; 9: 76.

Shepherd J. Private school applicants have a better change of getting into medical school. *The Guardian*, Wednesday 5 August 2009.

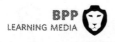

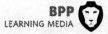

Chapter 3

An overview of Graduate Entry Medicine

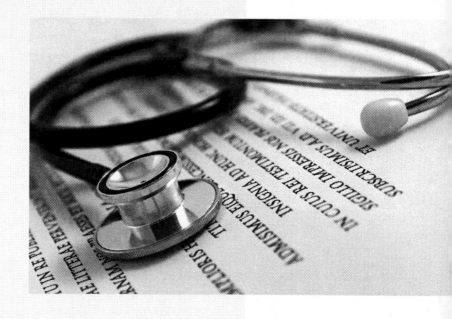

An overview of Graduate Entry Medicine

As described in the previous chapter, there are several routes through which graduates may gain entrance to study Medicine in the UK. Of these routes, it is the shortened Graduate Entry Medicine course that remains the most elusive to prospective applicants, and the purpose of this chapter is to provide you with an overview of the main components that comprise most Graduate Entry Medicine courses.

For entry in 2012, the GMC has approved 16 Graduate Entry Medicine courses, comprehensive details of which are provided in Chapter 4. Each of the 16 medical schools offering Graduate Entry Medicine courses are unique and differ with respect to eligibility, content and delivery. Given this variation, the prospect of selecting the right course for you can seem quite daunting, however, there are several common elements that help to distinguish (and unite) graduate entry students from their undergraduate counterparts. Indeed, accreditation by the GMC, which is a requirement for all medical courses in the UK, is itself a source of governance that serves to ensure that Graduate Entry Medicine entrants meet the same basic outcome criteria of all newly qualified doctors. Details of these outcome measures are outlined in the document *Tomorrow's Doctors*.

Having made the difficult decision to study Graduate Entry Medicine, the next major hurdles are to identify, apply to and secure a place of study. Each medical school sets its own admission criteria, which partly reveals the nature of the course, since the teaching style of any Graduate Entry Medicine course will reflect the type of graduate they accept. For example, certain medical schools, such as the University of Oxford require a degree in a Science or health-related subject, while other medical schools, such as the University of Nottingham, accept graduates from any subject area, including the Arts and Humanities. As a general rule, the broader the range of degree subjects accepted, the greater the proportion of traditional, didactic learning that is taught. In contrast, courses which require Science or health-related degree subjects tend to have a greater proportion of problem-based learning (PBL). It should be emphasised that this loose generalisation becomes increasingly less relevant after the first 12 to 18 months, as in most instances students then integrate with their undergraduate colleagues.

Course structure

Traditionally, undergraduate medical education has been split into two stages: first, during the pre-clinical stage, students develop their knowledge and understanding of the basic sciences, largely within the confines of the medical school. Second, during the clinical stage, learning is focused on the diagnosis and management of different disease states. Students still receive teaching at Medical School during the clinical stage, albeit to a much lesser extent than during the pre-clinical stage. Instead, most teaching is received on placement at local hospitals and primary care practices. For undergraduate courses, the pre-clinical stage lasts two to three years, and the clinical stage typically lasts three years.

The fundamental difference between Graduate Entry Medicine and Undergraduate Medicine is the course duration, with Graduate Entry Medicine taking one year less than the standard undergraduate degree. With a shorter training period, several factors contribute to ensuring that Graduate Entry Medicine students meet the same outcome measures as their undergraduate colleagues. These include:

- Graduates bring with them a range of prior skills and experiences that form the foundation for further learning.
- A problem-based approach to study.
- A greater requirement for self-directed study.
- An emphasis on inter-professional learning.
- Early clinical contact from year one.

In terms of structure, most Graduate Entry Medicine courses incorporate an accelerated phase where aspects of the undergraduate course are covered in a shorter period of time. The most common approach is to cover the pre-clinical stage of the course in 12 to 18 months, rather than the two years on the undergraduate course. This is typically followed by integration with the undergraduate course for the clinical stage. The accelerated period of study can be an extremely intense time for Graduate Entry Medicine students, due to the large volume of demanding material to be covered over a short period of time. Consequently, motivation and an affinity

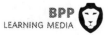

for self-directed study are two characteristics that are particularly important during this challenging period of study.

Learning style

Each of the 16 Graduate Entry Medicine courses contain an element of teaching distinct from the traditional models of didactic lecturing where the emphasis is on diligent note taking and rote learning. Specific forms of learning you are likely to encounter on the Graduate Entry Medicine course include PBL, integrated learning, inter-professional learning, and self-directed learning. Some of these learning styles will be familiar to you from your previous undergraduate experiences, while others are likely to be completely new. It should be appreciated that while described individually, it is more common (and often more effective) to find aspects of each being used simultaneously. This development is not unique to Graduate Entry Medicine courses as traditional models of learning have also been reduced in the undergraduate curricula across all medical schools in the UK, albeit to a lesser extent.

Foremost among the learning styles of a Graduate Entry Medicine course is PBL. During a PBL session, graduates work in small groups on clinical cases or scenarios. The PBL model works on the principle that the knowledge of the group is greater than that of any one individual and an emphasis is placed on collaboration between group members through the sharing of information and experiences. The Graduate Entry Medicine cohort will, by definition, comprise individuals with a variety of degree subjects, including Biomedical Science, Biochemistry, Pharmacy, Biology, Psychology, and Nursing, to name but a few. In the context of Graduate Entry Medicine, it makes practical sense that the efforts of this diverse group of students are best served by an integrated approach, allowing individuals to learn from one another in a more comprehensive and efficient way.

In general, traditional learning practices are minimal, and may even be actively discouraged at certain medical schools, such as the taking of notes during PBL sessions, as this may detract from the productivity of the group. Instead, individuals are encouraged to discuss ideas and share information. Typically, at the beginning of a PBL session a case scenario is introduced and is used as a discussion tool from which learning objectives are developed.

Students subsequently undertake self-directed learning before returning to the group to share their findings. In the context of small groups, PBL assists in the development of core competencies such as:

- Communication skills.
- Responsibility for one's own learning.
- Tolerance of others.
- Effective time management.
- Confidence, independence and initiative.

Difficult topics may be supplemented with lectures or complementary resources, such as small group tutorials, thus providing a link between PBL and the traditional models of teaching. Teachers adopt a facilitatory role, providing input to a group when additional guidance or support is required and providing feedback, which is an important tool for continued professional development.

Problem-based learning: how does it work?

Several models of PBL exist; however, they are all derived from a system first developed at McMaster University Medical School, Canada, during the 1960s.

Each PBL session consists of a group of students, usually between eight and ten, and a facilitator (otherwise known as a moderator). Within the PBL group, students nominate a person to act as chair for the session, as well as a scribe to capture salient information, usually on a whiteboard. PBL modules are usually broken down into individual scenarios, and groups typically remain together for the duration of the module. This serves two purposes: firstly, it allows for the development of group dynamics and secondly, it allows for the rotation of the positions of chair and scribe between members of the group.

Today, many medical schools in the UK have adopted a system known as the 'Maastricht seven step' process, which proceeds as follows:

1.	The group reads through the PBL scenario and clarifies any unfamiliar terms. The scribe makes note of any terms that remain uncertain.

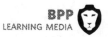

2. The group makes a brief summary of what they believe the problem is and the scribe makes a record of this.

3. The group discusses the problem and provides preliminary explanations based on their prior knowledge. The scribe captures ideas via a mind-map or brainstorm.

4. The group reviews the work and begins to prioritise information. The scribe may highlight specific information to return to in a later session.

5. The group devises learning objectives (usually between 10 and 15). This is often a challenging part of the session and the facilitator may need to provide guidance, particularly for groups new to the PBL process. The scribe may publish these for the group, via an intranet or email system.

6. Individuals from the group attempt to complete the learning objectives in preparation for the next session where they will share information with the rest of the group.

7. The group reconvenes to share their findings while the facilitator ensures that the learning objectives have been met.

To illustrate a typical week of PBL, the following example is taken from the University of Birmingham graduate entry course. PBL groups meet on a Tuesday morning to discuss a new scenario. Over the course of several hours the group works through steps 1 to 5 of the Maastricht process, as described above, concluding the session by devising a set of learning objectives. The role of the facilitator is to ensure that the learning objectives devised reflect those of the curriculum while ensuring the group remains on task. Each group member then individually reviews the learning objectives before the next meeting on Friday, when the group, led by the chair, discuss each learning objective in turn. The second PBL session is an opportunity to share information and identify any areas for further learning or clarification. The group then reconvene on the following Tuesday to review any outstanding points from the preceding PBL scenario before commencing the next scenario. At this point, the roles of chair and scribe are rotated.

Individual PBL scenarios are grouped into blocks lasting several weeks, with each block constituting a 'module'. At the end of the module the group members may be changed, or they may continue through a further module together. The exact duration of a PBL session, scenario, or module will vary between institutions, as will the length of time the group remains together.

PBL and your application

There are some important considerations regarding the course learning style to think about when short-listing medical schools to apply. These include:

- How much of the course is delivered using PBL?
- Does PBL suit your learning style?
- What additional resources are used to supplement PBL? For example, small group tutorials, supplementary lectures, or study workbooks.

What are the challenges of PBL?

PBL can present Graduate Entry Medicine students with unique challenges. A fortunate few will have experience of the process from their previous studies, or professional careers, however the majority will have no experience of PBL whatsoever. The new learning environment is extremely challenging, particularly since the volume of work at times may seem overwhelming. Often these feelings are greatest at the beginning, when the group are least familiar with one another and confidence in the PBL process is at its lowest. Over time, and with the support of the group facilitators, the PBL process becomes second nature.

As with any group, a range of individual characteristics and personalities will exist. This in itself can present challenges; particularly when there are clashes of opinion, or when individuals adopt a particularly passive, or assertive role. Indeed, this highlights the point that PBL requires a greater amount of individual participation in comparison to courses that are largely lectured-based. Moreover, the learning objectives of each scenario are determined by the group, and responsibility for covering the required content, the extent and depth of which is unspecified, lies with the individual. Contrast this with traditional lecture-based courses, where material is provided in a structured format and delivered by knowledgeable and experienced teachers, and it is clear that PBL requires a more independent and mature approach to learning.

Integrated versus traditional curricula

A traditional medical curriculum is one that covers subjects such as Physiology, Anatomy and Neuroscience individually. This approach has, until recently, been the main way in which the pre-clinical years of a medical degree have been taught. In contrast to this, an integrated curriculum is one that focuses on the interdisciplinary nature of Medicine. With an integrated approach, you do not learn the anatomy and physiology of organs (for example, the kidney) in isolation, but rather the whole system (in this instance, the renal system). In doing so, it may be necessary to study the blood supply to the organ, thus introducing study of the vascular system. This is an example of horizontal integration, whereby medical disciplines are covered alongside one another, and has become increasingly popular amongst medical schools. This approach seeks to build upon prior knowledge, which until recently has largely been the preserve of the clinical years.

As outlined, Graduate Entry Medicine courses tend to introduce clinical contact from an earlier stage (and often from the outset), thus further blurring the distinction between the pre-clinical and clinical years. This approach is potentially better suited to Graduate Entry Medicine courses as prior academic, professional and life experiences are likely to equip the graduate student for earlier 'vertical' integration.

Integrating with the undergraduate course

With the exception of the University of Warwick and the University of Swansea, which operate purely graduate entry courses, all Graduate Entry Medicine students integrate with their undergraduate colleagues at some point. As described above, for most courses this occurs after an accelerated phase on the Graduate Entry Medicine course. Integration of graduate entry students with their undergraduate counterparts usually occurs at the junction between the pre-clinical and clinical years of the course. Once integrated, Graduate Entry Medicine students follow a curriculum that is closely aligned to the undergraduate curriculum with the addition or removal of certain aspects to provide a more tailored syllabus.

These nuances may be reflected by differences in some of the formal assessment between the courses, or the types of optional modules that are available. As the clinical years proceed, integration becomes more complete and individual differences between the graduate entry and undergraduate curricula may disappear altogether.

Aside from the academic differences, there are other implications of the integration between the Graduate Entry Medicine and undergraduate courses. The introduction of a new group of 'older' students often raises questions by the undergraduate students about the nature of the graduate entry course. There are preconceptions on both sides: undergraduates often regard their older colleagues as over-zealous students, while graduate entry students may find their younger colleagues somewhat less enthusiastic learners than themselves. However, as integration of the two cohorts continues, the distinction between graduate and undergraduate students diminishes.

Intercalation

Unlike most other degree subjects, Medicine is unusual in that students are allowed to study for an additional degree, usually a BSc, as part of the core undergraduate training. The GMC has identified two key objectives for students who intercalate. These are the development of research skills and the in-depth study of topics of interest to the student outside of the core medical syllabus. Generally, intercalation is undertaken as an additional year of study outside the medical curriculum and involves a research project in a Science subject. With the exception of a few medical schools that require every student to intercalate as part of a six-year undergraduate course, most allow students to apply to a restricted number of places. Given the natural juncture between the pre-clinical and clinical years, most undergraduate students tend to intercalate at this point. Since the majority of graduate entry courses consolidate the pre-clinical years into a one-year accelerated phase followed by integration with the 'principal' course, it is not surprising that it is at this stage when most Graduate Entry Medicine students, who wish to intercalate, choose to do so.

Advantages of intercalation as a Graduate Entry Medicine student

All Graduate Entry Medicine students will hold, as a minimum, a previous Bachelors degree, and many entrants will also hold a higher degree, such as a doctorate. In light of this, the option to study for an additional degree may not immediately seem relevant, however, many of the benefits of undertaking an intercalated degree are still relevant to Graduate Entry Medicine students, particularly those who do not hold degrees in the Sciences, or allied health professions. Furthermore, some medical schools allow students on graduate entry courses to study towards a Masters, rather than a Bachelors degree, thus providing the attractive proposition of attaining a higher degree. Reasons to intercalate cited by Graduate Entry Medicine students include:

- The desire to broaden one's experience in a subject or topic that is distinct from their previous degree.
- The acquisition of a Science-related degree where one is not previously held.
- Having an interest in a subject that is likely to form part of a future career specialty.
- Having a strong interest in academia and research.
- The opportunity to develop new skills in areas such as research, analysis, project management and essay writing.
- Intercalation may further distinguish applicants thus providing opportunities for faster progression up the career ladder.

Disadvantages of intercalation as a Graduate Entry Medicine student

There are a number of implications to consider when contemplating intercalation. Factors common to graduate entry and undergraduate students include:

- Adding an additional year of study to an already lengthy degree.
- The financial burden of an additional year of study.
- Medical schools often require students to achieve grades above a certain threshold; Graduate Entry Medicine students may find this particularly challenging due to the accelerated nature of the course.

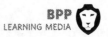

In addition, factors specific to Graduate Entry Medicine students include:

- Graduate Entry Medicine students are likely to carry a greater burden of existing financial debt and may not be able to afford to intercalate.
- Only one additional degree can be included on the Foundation Programme application form when applying for a Foundation Year 1 doctor role, thus negating the value of holding multiple Bachelors degrees.

Having weighed up the advantages and disadvantages of intercalation, there are also additional factors specific to each medical school that must be considered. It is important to note that these are not unique to graduate students, but instead are relevant to any student considering intercalation.

Foremost is to ensure that you identify the right course for you. Following the introduction of integrated curricula, the variety of courses offered by the various medical schools has increased dramatically with most schools accepting both internal and external applicants. Consequently, should you find a different medical school offers your ideal course, it is worthwhile enquiring whether you are able to apply as an external applicant. At this time, it may also be helpful to speak with a career adviser, or tutor, who can provide you with relevant and up to date information.

Having found the ideal course, it is important to gain a clear understanding of what will be expected of you before and after you start the course. An ideal place to find out is through students who are currently undertaking, or have recently completed the course you are interested in. Course supervisors, lecturers and department leads are also an excellent source of information.

The medical elective

The medical elective is traditionally offered as part of the core curriculum at most medical courses and for the majority of Graduate Entry Medicine courses it is completed at the end of the penultimate, or start of the final year. This period of study, which usually lasts between three to twelve weeks, represents an opportunity to pursue an area of personal interest as well as develop and use skills in

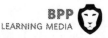

research, reflection, planning and organisation. For this reason the elective is also referred to as a Student-Selected Component (SSC). Many students decide to undertake their elective abroad and gain experience of different cultures, societies and health systems, while others decide to study closer to home. Wherever the elective is undertaken, its purpose is to provide experience of healthcare provision in a different environment.

In the document *Tomorrow's Doctors* the GMC identifies six goals for all SSCs, including the elective:

1. Learn about and begin to develop and use research skills.
2. Have greater control over their own learning and develop self-directed learning skills.
3. Study, in depth, topics of particular interest outside the core curriculum.
4. Develop greater confidence in their own skills and abilities.
5. Present the results of their work verbally, visually or in writing.
6. Consider potential career paths.

Each medical school provides its own guidelines regarding the organisation of the elective and a comprehensive overview is beyond the scope of this book. However, as a starting point to help you gain the most from your elective it is important to consider the following:

*   What topic or area do you want to look at during your elective? This is likely to reflect both your personal and professional interests.
*   What do you hope to gain from your elective experience? Examples include life experiences, travel, experience of different healthcare systems or academic and professional development.
*   What contribution can you make to the area and people you are visiting?
*   Are there any ethical, safety or political considerations about the area you plan to visit?
*   What are the financial implications of your chosen elective and are these justifiable?

- How can you best prepare for the elective? Most students have to produce a reflective report about their experiences and previous reports, presentations, and essays on the area of your elective are an excellent source of information.

The above list is by no means exhaustive. Often you will be expected to identify a supervisor, typically a clinician or academic within the medical school to whom you will make a proposal for your elective topic. If you study away from your medical school you will be required to identify a supervisor at the elective location as well, and this person may be able to provide you with practical information relating to accommodation and travel. As described above, most schools will require you to produce a report as a means of formal assessment. Above all else, the elective represents an opportunity to gain practical experience in an area of Medicine that interests you. Good planning, organisation and a proactive approach will ensure that you obtain the most out of your placement.

 Summary

- Several routes of entry are available to the graduate student seeking to study Medicine.
- One route that has become increasingly popular (and competitive) is the four-year Graduate Entry Medicine course.
- Most Graduate Entry Medicine courses include an accelerated period of study that lasts for 12 to 18 months and is equivalent to the preclinical period of undergraduate course.
- During the accelerated period Graduate Entry Medicine courses typically include a greater proportion of modern teaching methods, compared to their undergraduate equivalents
- Modern teaching methods include PBL, integrated learning and self-directed learning.
- With the exception of medical schools providing only Graduate Entry Medicine, integration of graduate entry students with their undergraduate colleagues blurs the distinction between the two cohorts during the latter years of the course.

- On completion of the course, Graduate Entry Medicine students achieve the same basic outcome criteria and clinical skills as undergraduate medical students. This allows them to apply for the Foundation Programme, which represents the start of their professional career.

 Useful resources

www.gmc-uk.org/education (*Tomorrow's Doctors*)
www.bma.org.uk
www.foundationprogramme.nhs.uk
Wood DF ABC of learning and teaching in medicine. Problem based learning. *BMJ* 2003; 326(8): 328–330.

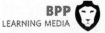

Chapter 4

Choosing a
Medical School

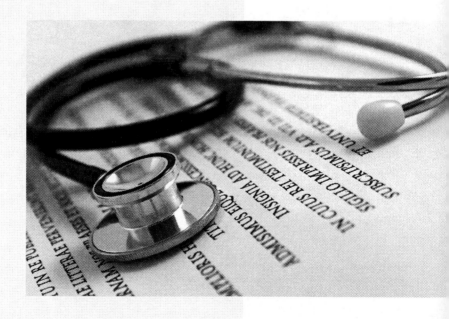

Choosing a Medical School

Introduction

This chapter provides an overview of the 16 Graduate Entry Medicine courses that currently exist in the UK. The chapter focuses upon key aspects of each course, helping you to decide between the different medical schools. In addition, a major feature of this chapter is the inclusion of students reviews from those currently studying on each of the graduate entry courses.

University and course description

There are several criteria that you may wish to consider when making your choice of medical schools. To help you make this decision, this chapter includes information for each medical school regarding degree courses accepted and academic requirements, intake per year, applicants per place and the selection process. In addition, the course structure is described in terms of the teaching style, integration with the undergraduate course, transition from pre-clinical to clinical medicine, hospital attachments and elective placements.

Course ranking

Furthermore, for each medical school, you will find the school's ranking for the academic year 2012 according to the 'The Complete University Guide' (*The Independent*). The ranking takes into account the following four factors: student satisfaction, graduate prospects, quality of research and entry standards. This ranking system includes every medical school in the UK, including those which do not offer Graduate Entry Medicine. Furthermore, the scores are based on the overall performance of the medical school, thereby incorporating both the Undergraduate and Graduate Entry Medicine courses where they are both offered.

Before reading the sections that follow, it is important to note that many components of the medical degrees offered are either similar, or identical across the UK due to the requirements set by the GMC. Firstly, all courses will feature clinical placements in primary (mostly GP practices) and secondary care (mostly hospitals); these commence at varying stages in different schools, but almost

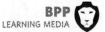

all graduate courses introduce clinical placements in the first year. While the student-to-consultant ratio, time spent in each specialty and facilities of the hospitals differ slightly, all universities are required to produce foundation-year doctors that meet a certain standard and thus the clinical phase of the 16 medical schools show fewer differences compared to many other university courses.

Another example of the similarity between courses is the SSC, whereby students are able to pursue a subject of interest over a set period. Again, every medical school offers these, however many of the graduate entry courses do not contain these components in the first year. Most courses also involve learning several non-scientific subjects, such as Ethics, Law, Sociology, and Communication Skills.

Also, many of the entry requirements are shared between medical schools, such as evidence of work experience, proof of immunisation against certain diseases, a CRB (Criminal Record Bureau) check and agreement to sign a student declaration of some form. Some medical schools do not accept applications from students who are yet to complete their bachelor degree and most medical schools reject UCAS applications for deferred entry.

Student review

When choosing a course it is often valuable to find out what it is like to study from a students' perspective. Therefore, to allow you to gain a deeper understanding of each of the courses from a medical student's point of view the chapter also includes a review of each of the courses by students currently on the course. Students were asked to comment on the course, the medical school and university, as well as the local area.

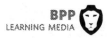

Medical schools

Barts and The London

- **Courses accepted**: Bachelors degree in a science or health related discipline.
- **Academic requirements**: A first or upper second (2:1) class Honours degree or an equivalent European/overseas qualification. A first class Masters is accepted in place of a second class Bachelor degree. AS level Chemistry and Biology at grade A or B, or equivalent are required. The website provides additional information on the entry requirements.
- **Total intake per year**: 40
- **Applicants per place**: 24
- **Selection process**: UKCAT followed by an assessment centre based interview (takes place in February). This interview involves a written exercise, commenting on a doctor-patient consultation or similar, a teamwork exercise and completion of a questionnaire.

University and course description

Barts and The London School of Medicine and Dentistry is the Medical School of the Queen Mary University in London, and was formed in 1995 from the merger of the Medical College of St Bartholomew's Hospital and The London Hospital Medical College. Of the London universities, the Queen Mary differs from many others in offering principally campus-based facilities. As with its undergraduate programme, the graduate entry pre-clinical phase follows a problem-based learning (PBL) system of learning in groups of eight to ten students and lasts for one year. Patient contact occurs in the first year through community-based placements in general practices. The clinical phase comprises years two to four and is integrated with the undergraduate course. During these years, lectures continue and tutorials are based on real-life situations. Teaching occurs at three sites: the Whitechapel (site of the Royal London Hospital), Mile End Campus and the City of London. Clinical placements occur in the Royal London and Barts hospitals, Homerton Hospital, Newham General and

Whipps Cross University Hospital, as well as other hospitals in Greater London and Essex. The elective occurs following successful completion of the final examinations. The Barts and The London School of Medicine and Dentistry was ranked 6th in the Complete University Guide league table.

Student review

The course

The first year combines years one and two of the standard five-year course. The first year of the course encompasses PBL with supplementary lectures. Clinical contact is provided by regular alternate visits at a hospital or GP practice. The geographic location of hospitals for the clinical years range from central London going eastwards towards Southend. Prosections aid anatomy teaching. The course is very intense and a lot work is required to pass the tests at the end of each module and at the end of the year. A feature of the course is studying alongside graduate entry nurses. Students come from a variety of backgrounds, which is useful in different aspects of the course and being a small group of around 40, you develop friends for life.

The medical school/university

The medical school is situated at Whitechapel and Barbican tube stations. The Royal London Hospital is due to move to a new building in 2012, which will provide superior medical and teaching facilities. Barts has already undergone major renovations. The medical school is very receptive to ideas from its students and is keen to attempt to implement or change to provide a better experience for its students. The location of the medical school provides excellent exposure to certain conditions, such as TB, that are rarely seen elsewhere in the country. During the first year, every Wednesday afternoon is dedicated to sports time or social activities and is always free from lectures. The medical school also has a great reputation for raising money for various charities.

The local area

Most students choose to live in East London owing to the availability of affordable accommodation and excellent transport links to placements and the City. However, it is possible to live anywhere

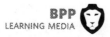

in London. The student union has a regular programme of events that are well attended, and the bright lights of London are only a short journey away.

University accommodation is available for first-year students, and is based close to St Bartholemew's hospital in Charterhouse Square. This large accommodation block has a bar and gym on site, and is well served by bus, tube and rail links. Further accommodation is available in Whitechapel and Mile End. During the middle years of the course, many students choose to live together in large student houses.

Additional information

- Website address: www.smd.qmul.ac.uk/admissions/ Medicine/gep
- Contact details
  Barts and The London School of Medicine & Dentistry
  Garrod Building
  Turner Street
  Whitechapel
  London
  E1 2AD
  gepmedicine@qmul.ac.uk

University of Birmingham

- **Courses accepted**: Biochemistry, Biological Sciences*, Biomedical Science, Dentistry, Human Biology, Medical Biochemistry, Nursing*, Pharmacology, Pharmacy, Physiology, Physiotherapy, Podiatry, Psychology*, Sports Science*, and Sports Studies*.
- **Academic requirements**: A first or upper second class (2:1) Honours degree. In practice, only those with first-class Honours degrees are accepted. Knowledge of Chemistry is also required (equivalent to a grade C or better at A level).
- **Total intake per year**: 40
- **Applicants per place**: 11
- **Selection process**: Structured interview only, there are no admission tests at present.

* Dependent on syllabus. Contact the medical school for verification.

University and course description

The graduate programme at the University of Birmingham has been running since 2002. The pre-clinical phase of the Birmingham course takes place during the first year, in which learning occurs within a PBL framework with some additional lectures. Patient contact begins in the first year with a weekly placement in a GP surgery. The remaining three years make up the clinical phase, and are integrated with the principal (five-year) course. The second year consists of two 10-week placements in general Medicine and Surgery, while years three and four consist of rotations in more specialist areas. Placements during the clinical years are usually within a ten mile radius of the medical school and accessible using Birmingham's extensive transport system. The furthest placement is Hereford, although few students are allocated there and on-site accommodation is available. In line with most medical schools, the course involves an elective period; this lasts for five weeks and occurs within an eight-week window in the penultimate year. The Birmingham medical school was ranked 7th overall in the Complete University Guide league table.

Student review

The course

The Birmingham course consists of a one-year accelerated pre-clinical course, after which students integrate with the principal course students for three clinical years which are largely based in hospitals and GP particles in Birmingham and the surrounding area. The first year of the course is predominantly PBL which involves a large component of self-directed learning and consequently requires a fair degree of self motivation. A typical week includes two group meetings to discuss the week's PBL topic; an 'experts' session with a subject specialist to discuss the week's topic in more detail, a day of community based medicine at a local GP practice, an afternoon of anatomy teaching using plastic models and prosections, in addition to approximately four hours of lectures. Students come from a range of backgrounds, however, the majority arrive with some form of Bioscience degree. Being the only course

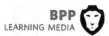

of its kind requiring a first class honours degree, students tend to be academic and hard working.

The medical school/university

The medical school is situated in the leafy suburbs of Edgbaston. As one of the largest medical schools in the country, it boasts an extensive medical library, a new prosectorium, a large computer cluster and the 450 seat Leonard Deacon lecture theatre. The main campus, situated opposite the Medical School, is composed of red brick Victorian buildings set around the central clock tower. In the first year of the course, graduate students are predominantly based in a one of four PBL rooms which are equipped with key textbooks, anatomical models and computer facilities. Around half of the clinical placements are a short distance from the medical school. A car, while highly advantageous for distant placements, is not a necessity. There are a large range of sports clubs and societies offered by the medical school that cater for most tastes and have the advantage of being geared around the medical student timetable.

The local area

The majority of graduate entry students live in the village of Harborne, a 15-minute walk from the university, known for its choice of restaurants and the 'pub mile'. Other popular areas include Selly Oak, where the university is based, well served by local shops, supermarkets, restaurants and pubs. Some students choose to live in the city centre, which is within a ten-minute drive. The University of Birmingham is the only university to be served by its own train station that provides a direct link to the city centre. As the country's second city, Birmingham has a huge range of nightlife activities to suit every taste, from the large popular clubs on Broad Street, to the smaller bars and pubs in the historic Jewellery Quarter, Moseley and Brindley Place. Those who take shopping seriously are well served by the UK's busiest shopping centre, the Bullring, and vintage shops in Digbeth. Birmingham is a highly multi-cultural city, housing several art galleries, food from every continent, and the famous 'Balti triangle'.

Additional information

- Website address: www.medicine.bham.ac.uk/ug/gec
- Contact details:
  Medical School
  College of Medical and Dental Science
  University of Birmingham
  Edgbaston
  Birmingham
  B15 2TT
  Email: mdsenquiries@contacts.bham.ac.uk

University of Bristol

- **Courses accepted**: Those under the broad title of 'Medical Sciences': Anatomy, Biomedical Sciences, Cell Pathology, Dentistry, Neuroscience, Osteopathy, Pharmacology, Pharmacy, Physiology, and Physiotherapy. Biology, Biochemistry and Psychology that incorporate human science modules are also accepted.
- **Academic requirements**: A first or upper second (2:1) class Honours degree. Chemistry A level and one other science subject are also required. A grade B in Mathematics, English Language and two sciences at GCSE level are also required. Note that at least four months' of work experience as a Healthcare Assistant or similar are recommended by the university.
- **Total intake per year**: 19
- **Applicants per place**: 19
- **Selection process**: No admission test. Interviews held mid-November until the end of March. Note that candidates must complete an additional application form.

University and course description

The Graduate Entry Medicine course at the University of Bristol started in 2006 and is one of the smallest in the UK. The pre-clinical phase occurs in the first year, thereafter students integrate with the undergraduate course. The first year is an amalgamation of years one and two of the undergraduate course, however all graduate students are required to undertake the 'Molecular and Cellular Basis of Medicine' module and may be able to omit some

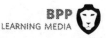

anatomy modules depending on their educational background. Unlike PBL-based courses, teaching focuses more upon lectures, practical classes and small-group teaching. Patient contact occurs in the first year with placements in a general practice clinic. The remainder of the course involves several clinical placements, with an opportunity for an elective in the final year of the course. The Bristol medical school was ranked 19th overall in the Complete University Guide league table.

Student review

The course

The Bristol course consists of one pre-clinical year where students are immediately integrated into the five-year course. In this year, students attend the second year systems-based lecture programme with a one-week clinical attachment after each system taught. Where possible, students also attend first year lectures on the human basis of Medicine. The majority of teaching follows a traditional lecture based learning style. There can be clashes in the programme for graduate students that may require a degree of organisation and flexibility, however, most students do not have any trouble with this. Students typically accepted have a minimum of an upper second class degree in a human bioscience subject and some relevant work experience. The final three years of the course are based in the Clinical Academies spread throughout the Severn Deanery. During these years, graduate students follow the same programme as the principal five-year course. Students are provided with accommodation if the Academy is outside of Bristol.

The medical school/university

The medical school is central to the university, situated between the city centre and Clifton. The majority of the pre-clinical year is based around two lecture theatres and the anatomy department on St Michael's Hill. The anatomy department is one of the few in the country to continue to teach using cadaver-based prosection. The Clinical Academies are based in Somerset, North Bristol, South Bristol, Weston-Super-Mare, Gloucestershire and Bath. Each of these have clinical skills labs allowing you to work in a range of clinical environments in smaller groups. Bristol also offers an ERASMUS programme where students can opt to exchange to train in a range of European cities for a semester where they can improve language

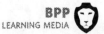

skills and experience a different educational environment. Galenicals is the University of Bristol's Medical Student society which boasts 12 sports teams, music, drama, its own magazine and many socials throughout the academic year.

The local area

Student halls of residence are a 40-minute walk from St Michael's Hill, but many students live in the suburbs of Clifton, Redland, Cotham and Kingsdown. The city centre is rarely more than walking distance and contains great opportunities for shopping and eating in Broadmead, the new Cabot Circus shopping centre and the waterfront. There is a buzzing nightlife with something for all tastes from the mainstream bars and clubs of Clifton triangle, to the street art, music and independent shops of Stokes Croft. Bristol, famous for Banksy, balloons and bridges, is full of character and culture that you will inevitably fall in love with, one of Briton's truly remarkable cities.

Additional information

*   Website address: www.bris.ac.uk/medical-school/prospective-students/graduate
*   Contact details:
    Medical Admissions Assistant
    Faculty of Medicine and Dentistry
    69 St Michael's Hill
    Bristol
    BS2 8DZ
    Email: med-admissions@bristol.ac.uk

University of Cambridge

*   **Courses accepted**: All degree disciplines are accepted.
*   **Academic requirements**: A first or upper second (2:1) class Honours degree, as well as A level Chemistry with passes at AS or A levels in two of Physics, Biology or Mathematics. Grade C or above is also required in Double Award Science and Mathematics at GSCE level; GCSE Biology and Physics may be substituted for Double Award Science. Please note that candidates are required to complete a separate application form specific to Cambridge.

- **Total intake per year**: 20
- **Applicants per place**: 8
- **Selection process**: Candidates may opt to take the BMAT (Biomedical Aptitude Test) to meet pre-medical requirements; candidates with successful applications are interviewed.

University and course description

Applications to Cambridge (as well as Oxford) vary slightly from other institutions in the UK, partly due to its division into colleges. Firstly, Cambridge administers an extra charge known as the 'college fee' that amounts approximately to £5,000; this is paid annually in addition to the tuition fee, although your chosen college may pay this on your behalf (please visit the University of Cambridge website for the latest information). For those eligible for an NHS bursary, this covers the college fee from years two to four of the course. Applicants can apply to a specific college at Cambridge, or submit an open application. College preference should not advantage or prejudice an application in any way, but colleges do vary in age, size, location and student population (for example, some are graduate-only colleges). Teaching is largely standardised across the colleges as most teaching occurs centrally. Currently three colleges at Cambridge offer places in Graduate Medicine: Hughes Hall, Lucy Cavendish (female students only) and Wolfson College. For Graduate Entry Medicine, candidates are able to apply to both Oxford and Cambridge in the same academic year.

The Cambridge graduate course, which first started in 2005, adopts a problem-solving approach that involves weekly supervisions (tutorial-based sessions) and lectures. Pre-clinical and clinical phases of the course are closely integrated; with the basic science modules of the pre-clinical phase taking place over the first 20 months. Students also attend four clinical placements during this initial period. These placements occur during the vacations in the West Suffolk area, and involve one and a half days a week in general practice and the remaining days in hospital. The core medical sciences units are drawn from the first four and a half terms of the standard undergraduate course, and graduates are required to sit the same exams. The final two years of the course are entirely clinical and involve further supervisions from clinical doctors. Clinical placements take place in Addenbrooke's and other teaching hospitals in the regions of East Anglia and the South East.

The elective occurs in the summer of the third year. The Cambridge Medical School was ranked 4th overall in the Complete University Guide league table.

There is an additional route of entry to Medicine, unique to the University of Cambridge , which is known as the 'affiliate' course. This enables graduates to take the undergraduate course (usually lasting six-years) with omission of the third year. Three colleges currently offer this option (Lucy Cavendish, St Edmund's and Wolfson) and NHS funding is only available for the final year.

Student review

The course

The first two years of the course are lecture based, with hospital experience commencing after the eight-week term where students put core sciences into context – for example, in the first year, after covering Cardiac Physiology and Anatomy, students spend time in the Cardiology department. The final two 'clinical years' involve eight-week rotations in the various medical and surgical specialties (including Obstetrics and Gynaecology, Paediatrics, Neurology, Rheumatology, Orthopaedics and Psychiatry) and include a two-week placement in General Practice at the end of each rotation. These years require a more proactive self-directed approach with an emphasis on close interaction with patients. The graduate course covers the same core material as the standard course; with students even attending the same lectures and labs as the standard course students, but as the graduate entry course is small, it is a close-knit, highly supportive group. Furthermore, students come from a wide range of academic backgrounds, from degrees in English or Russian through to Astrophysics and Biochemistry.

The medical school/university

The facilities at the medical school are second to none. As the graduate entry course is small, students essentially get the whole of West Suffolk Hospital for the majority of the course, giving easy access to attend ward rounds and clinics, and most of the consultants know the students by their first names! Furthermore, the distance to clinical placements is immaterial because there is free hospital accommodation for placements away from Cambridge. Cambridge is one of the oldest and most historic universities, full

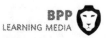

of beautiful architecture, and divided into colleges, though only three offer Graduate Entry Medicine. Most nightlife takes place in the colleges which have their own bars, and in terms of social life, there is a strong history of sports at Cambridge, with a particular rivalry against Oxford, especially in boating and rugby.

The local area

Cambridge is a university town, with 20% of residents being students! As a city it is full of beauty and history, with stunning architecture, including its famous cobbled streets. Most people choose to cycle around Cambridge, one of the UK's 11 'cycling cities' and you can easily hire bikes to get around if you choose not to buy one. When it comes to things to do, there are outdoor public tennis courts, an outdoor swimming pool, theatres, the Corn Exchange and the Arts Theatre. There are also plenty of gardens to stroll in – many attached to the colleges, the impressive Fitzwilliam Museum and the New Hall Art Collection for women-only artists. There are plenty of pubs and small clubs in Cambridge, and an abundance of independent shops and boutiques as well as high street stores, but if you want serious nightlife or shopping then London is less than an hour away on the train, with regular trains to Kings Cross and Liverpool St.

Additional information
- Website address: www.medschl.cam.ac.uk/education/courses/cgc
- Contact details:
  Cambridge Admissions Office
  University of Cambridge
  Fitzwilliam House
  32 Trumpington Street
  Cambridge
  CB2 1QY
  Email: admissions@cam.ac.uk

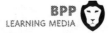

Imperial College London

- **Courses accepted**: Biological sciences related disciplines that incorporate a significant degree of Mammalian Physiology and Biochemistry. A formal checklist is available from the School's website, which should be validated by a tutor from your previous university.
- **Academic requirements**: A first or upper second (2:1) class Honours degree.
- **Total intake per year**: 50
- **Applicants per place**: 10
- **Selection process**: UKCAT followed by interview. Interviews usually take place in either late November or January.

University and course description

The Imperial College London course has been running since 2008, making it one of the most recent Graduate Entry Medicine courses to be developed. The first year of the course involves study of the pre-clinical modules in an accelerated form, in which material from the first two years of the standard six-year course is covered. Teaching takes various forms, including lectures, group tutorials and PBL. Clinical experience starts in the first year, with half a day spent each week on a clinical attachment. Following the first year, the Imperial graduate course merges with the undergraduate course for the clinical phase of the course. The elective takes place early in the spring term of the final year. The Imperial College Medical School was ranked 5th overall in the Complete University Guide league table.

Student review

The course

The Imperial course has an accelerated first year, after which students integrate fully with undergraduate students on the six-year course for clinical attachments. Most of the pre-clinical course is lecture based, focusing on Pathology, Physiology and Pharmacology in a systems based approach. The basic sciences are taught in small groups, along with self-directed study. One day per week is focused on Anatomy, which is taught with a combination of dissection, clinical laboratory sessions and lectures integrating new imaging techniques. There are also weekly PBL sessions. The clinical years

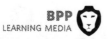

allow you to spend time in some of the top quaternary referral centres in the UK, such as Chelsea and Westminster and St Mary's hospitals. Students receive a mixture of central and peripheral site attachments, with the vast majority within the M25 and accessible via public transport. For those who prefer the District General Hospitals there are opportunities to swap placements to hospitals such as Hillingdon or St Peters.

The medical school/university

The first year of the course is based almost entirely at Hammersmith Hospital. This is half an hour from Charing Cross hospital where other medical students are based allowing the group to become well acquainted. Lectures are held in the newly renovated Wolfson Education Centre, where there is a common room with computer access, a canteen, a library and late opening study rooms. Imperial is one of the few medical schools to still have its own medical student's union based at the Charing Cross site, where most other student activities take place. With access to the main college union in South Kensington too, there is plenty to keep you busy! There are a huge number of clubs and societies for students, with a sports centre, swimming pools, gyms and squash courts at many of the hospital sites. Medical societies at Imperial form an important part of your time – with social and academic support from societies, through to revision lectures and mock exams set up by the medical education society.

The local area

In the first year, most students live near to the Hammersmith Hospital before moving closer to the Charing Cross site in Hammersmith. Hammersmith is well connected to both Central London and hospital sites across West London, enabling a balanced lifestyle. Accommodation is expensive and West London is one of the most expensive areas to live in the UK. Most students house share on arrival in London as accommodation in halls is currently not guaranteed for graduate students, however Imperial is currently developing a new campus with student accommodation close to the Hammersmith Hospital site. Socialising often takes the form of local pub quizzes, eating out, and the occasional formal dinner, though when students do choose to party there is something for everyone in London! West London is particularly well known for amazing shopping and there is much culture, with great music venues and museums and an increasingly thriving café culture.

Additional information

*   Website address: www1.imperial.ac.uk/medicine/teaching/undergraduate/ge
*   Contact details:
    School of Medicine Admissions
    Registry
    Imperial College London
    South Kensington campus
    London
    SW7 2AZ
    Email: medicine.ug.admissions@imperial.ac.uk

Keele University

*   **Courses accepted**: All degree subjects are accepted.
*   **Academic requirements**: A first or upper second (2:1) class Honours degree. GCSE English Language and Maths are required at grade C or above.
*   **Total intake per year**: 10
*   **Applicants per place**: 20
*   **Selection process**: GAMSAT followed by interview during December, February or March.

University and course description

The graduate programme at Keele University, with the smallest intake of all graduate entry courses, differs from many other medical schools in that graduates enter directly into the second year of the standard five-year course. Thus graduate students work alongside undergraduates from an early stage, with gaps in knowledge being filled by additional course content and self-directed learning. The PBL structure at Keele involves learning in groups of approximately 12 students, with a maximum of five to six supplementary lectures each week. Keele Medical School provides clinical exposure throughout the course, the first year involving placements in general practices as well as other clinical environments. Students learn in various hospitals throughout the

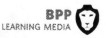
BPP
LEARNING MEDIA

course in and around Stafford, Shrewsbury and Telford, including the University Hospital of North Staffordshire (UHNS), and Shrewsbury and Telford Hospitals NHS Trust in Shropshire. The elective occurs in the final year of the Keele programme. Keele Medical School was ranked 30th overall in the Complete University Guide league table.

Student review

The course

At Keele, graduate entry students fully integrate with the undergraduate course during the first year. After two preparatory weeks, students join year two of the principal course. The course is well suited to those who prefer self-directed learning. Teaching takes the form of PBL in the first year of the graduate course. In subsequent years, group work is still integral to the learning process and takes the form of Case Based Learning and Case Informed Learning. Clinical placements take place within approximately a 30-mile radius. Most placements are accessible by public transport, and efforts are made to match clinical partners so that at least one has a car. Clinical placements commence in the first year, however become more intensive (four out of five days a week) in the second year and full-time in subsequent years. Placements are spread between Shrewsbury, North Staffordshire and Stafford hospitals.

The medical school/university

Keele Medical School is split between two buildings, one overlooking the main part of the university, and the other on the North Staffordshire Hospital site. There are additional teaching facilities on the other hospital sites in Shrewsbury and Stafford. The medical school at the Keele campus is well furbished with an anatomy suite, IT facilities, skills laboratories and a large lecture theatre. The hospital site houses the library, a wealth of smaller seminar rooms and purpose-built rooms for clinical skills. The experience of being a graduate medic at Keele is overwhelmingly inclusive. As the cohort of both graduate and five-year medics is small, it is possible to get to know the members of the medical school well – students and tutors alike. Problems are readily solved by the ease of liaison between members of the school. The discrete and easily accessed Student Support System allows more private or difficult issues to be discussed.

BPP
LEARNING MEDIA

The local area

As this is a Medical degree, it would be unrealistic to suggest that the average student enjoys boundless free time. However, it is important that recreation is built into the course, and all hobbies can be pursued through either the university or as part of the multitude of university or Medical societies. Nightlife is provided by the Union bar and by the nearby town centres of Newcastle and Hanley. Moreover, Manchester, Liverpool and Birmingham are within easy reach by train or car, and group hire of a minibus is affordable for visits to these cities. Keele University itself is a campus university, and is close to the town of Newcastle-under-Lyme. It is possible to live both on campus and in town in the first year, and students tend to live around the hospital sites in the remaining years.

Additional information

- Website address: http://www.keele.ac.uk/health/ schoolofmedicine/undergraduatemedicalcourse/ entryrouteshowtoapply/#a101
- Contact details:
  School of Medicine
  Admissions Office
  Keele University
  Staffordshire
  ST5 5BG
  Email: medadmissions@hfac.keele.ac.uk

King's College London

- **Courses accepted**: All degree subjects are accepted.
- **Academic requirements**: An upper second (2:1) class Honours degree is normally required, but a lower second (2:2) may be accepted if a candidate has a masters degree with at least a merit. Healthcare professionals without an honours degree may also be considered.
- **Total intake per year**: 24
- **Applicants per place**: 46
- **Selection process**: UKCAT followed by a structured interview with multiple stations.

University and course description

The King's College London graduate course has been running since 2004. The first year is a 'transition year', in which graduate students are taught pre-clinical based modules from the syllabus of years one and two of the standard course. The first year also includes some clinical exposure. Graduate students then proceed to join the third year of the standard five-year course. In the pre-clinical phase, teaching involves lectures and tutorials based at the Guy's Campus. The teaching is in a PBL format and case-based; it is partially shared with first and second year students from the five-year programme, the remainder being tailored to graduates. Learning usually occurs in small groups, except in clinical demonstrations and laboratory practicals where the entire cohort is taught together. The clinical phase of the course occurs in Guy's, King's Denmark Hill, and St Thomas' Hospitals. GP placements are typically in the London area, with some placements in University Hospital Lewisham, the South London and Maudsley NHS Foundation Trust and four District General Hospitals in the south-east (Ashford, Canterbury, Margate and Medway). The elective occurs in the final year. The King's College London Medical School was ranked 17th overall in the Complete University Guide league table.

Student review

The course

The first year is based at the Guy's Campus, and combines phases one and two of the five-year course, with integration onto the five-year course occurring in the second year. The first year involves much PBL and self-directed study, as well as demonstrations and practicals, which develops from the second year onwards to involve clinical placements and SSCs, and by the fourth year much time is spent on placements. Students come from a variety of academic backgrounds, including the Arts and as a result, the early stages cover the basic sciences. There is a strong emphasis on integrating clinical skills with teaching, therefore students have contact with patients from the first week of the course and progressively more in the second and latter years of the course. You also study alongside students from nursing and dentistry. There are plenty of facilities available for students including the new Simulation Centre, the Gordon Anatomy (pathology) Museum, a clinical skills centre with simulated wards, and two dissection rooms which are used regularly.

The medical school/university

The course is based across three central London hospital campuses; Guy's Hospital in London Bridge, St Thomas' Hospital near Waterloo and King's College Hospital, Denmark Hill, in South London, including 12 specialist centres and a network of over 300 general practices. The surrounding areas are densely populated, multi-ethnic and subject to high levels of disease, which means that the hospitals can provide students with the widest possible range of clinical experience. The university's facilities are second to none, with large libraries available at all three campuses (including the world famous Maughn Library in the Strand), and 24-hour computing facilities and study areas, a personal tutor, a support centre, health centre, and prayer facilities. All students have access to the King's College London Student Union, which has played host to a number of bands and consists of a huge range of societies including belly dancing, musical theatre and baking, and particular to medical students – Medecins sans Frontieres, Anaesthetic Society and Cardiology Society.

The local area

As the most central of London's universities, the campuses of King's College are well placed. The Denmark Hill Campus is near the Crystal Palace Stadium where a international athletics takes place, and Dulwich Picture Gallery, which is the oldest purpose-built public art gallery in England. The Guy's campus is minutes away from the fashionable South Bank area, where there are a number of restaurants and bars. Borough Market is also nearby – one of the oldest markets in the world. Finally, Waterloo Campus (including St. Thomas' Hospital) is next to London's South Bank, and not too far from the National Theatre and Royal Festival Hall. When it comes to living arrangements, the university has its own accommodation in the vicinity of these campuses, and there are also a large number of privately owned properties near the campuses, with a vast transport network of buses, tubes and trains to support students.

Additional information

- Website address: www.kcl.ac.uk/prospectus/undergraduate/ Medicine_graduate_professional_entry_programme
- Contact details:
  Student Admissions Office
  King's College London
  Guy's Campus
  London
  SE1 1UL
  Email: ug-healthadmissions@kcl.ac.uk

University of Leicester

- **Courses accepted**: All degree subjects accepted.
- **Academic requirements**: A first or upper second (2:1) class Honours degree. Also requires a minimum of one year of paid employment in a caring role.
- **Total intake per year**: 64
- **Applicants per place**: 10
- **Selection process**: UKCAT followed by interview.

University and course description

The University of Leicester graduate programme started in 2003 and is divided into Phases 1 and 2. Phase 1 lasts for 18 months, and takes place over three semesters during which time all pre-clinical and some clinical Medicine is covered. During the three semesters, graduates cover all the material from the standard five-year course. Phase 2 is the same as the undergraduate course and covers the remaining areas of clinical Medicine over two and a half years. Pre-clinical Medicine is taught via both lectures held with undergraduate students, and group work (typically of eight students). Group work includes some case studies and PBL, as well as presentations and other projects. Exposure to clinical Medicine occurs in the first phase, and includes hospital as well as general practice placements. The elective takes place in the final year of the course. The Leicester Medical School was ranked 15th overall in the Complete University Guide league table.

Student review

The course

The course is divided into two phases. Phase 1 consists of a combination of lectures, group work and clinical sessions in hospitals. Most lectures are with the five-year cohort and the group sessions require you to work through clinical scenarios in the module workbook in groups of eight. Each half day is dedicated to one module. A typical day may consist of a morning of lectures and small group sessions, followed by an afternoon of communication skills with a simulated patient. Phase 2 is split into several clinical placements, each lasting seven-weeks. On average, students spend half of these placements on 'out blocks', away from Leicester. Dissection plays a large part of the anatomy teaching at Leicester, with the added benefit of using whole body dissections.

The medical school/university

The medical school is situated next to a large park and the popular student area of Queens Road. It is also only a five-minute walk to the Leicester Royal Infirmary, where some clinical sessions and lectures take place. The university has a newly built library, in addition to the clinical sciences library at the Leicester Royal Infirmary, where every text book you could ever wish to read can be found. Students are allocated medic 'parents' who provide pastoral support, organise revision sessions and ensure social events are part of their 'children's' curriculum. 'LUSUMA' (Leicester's University Student's Union Medical Association) organises social, charity and sports events and aims to give medics a better university experience. There is a dedicated graduate representative who ensures that older students are not left out.

The local area

University halls are available and this is favoured by some students. However, in recent years, a popular approach for graduates has been to set up a Facebook group prior to the start of term and to arrange houses to rent together. Most medics live around the Clarendon Park area, which is within walking distance of the train station, medical school and perhaps more importantly, the bars and restaurants on Queens Road! The nightlife in Leicester may not compete with London, but it suits most needs. There are a range of pubs and clubs, and if you are interested in sport, the Leicester

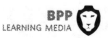

Tigers ground is only a short walk from campus. If shopping is more your scene, then the impressive Highcross shopping centre should curb any shopping cravings.

Additional information

- Website address: www.le.ac.uk/sm/le/
- Contact details:
  Graduate Admissions Tutor
  University of Leicester Medical School
  Maurice Shock Building
  PO Box 138
  University Road
  Leicester
  LE1 9HN
  Email: med-admis@le.ac.uk

University of Liverpool

- **Courses accepted**: Biomedical and health science degrees.
- **Academic requirements**: A first or upper second (2:1) class Honours degree, with an average of 65% or above, usually required. A levels: grades BBB or above, including A level Chemistry and Biology required. In addition, a minimum of nine GCSEs at Grade C are required.
- **Total intake per year**: 32
- **Applicants per place**: 12
- **Selection process**: No admissions tests required, offers are made following interview.

University and course description

The Liverpool Medical School runs medical courses as part of The Cumbria and Lancashire Medical and Dental Consortium, which consists of the University of Liverpool, Lancaster University, the University of Central Lancashire, and St Martin's College. While undergraduate courses are run at both the Universities of Liverpool and Lancaster, graduate courses are currently taken at the University of Liverpool only. The graduate programme was started in 2005. Like many other medical schools, the course includes an accelerated phase in the first year which covers the pre-clinical components of the first two years of the standard course. Thereafter, the Liverpool graduate cohort integrates fully with the principal course. Undergraduate and graduate teaching follows a PBL framework with early exposure to the clinical environment. Following completion of the first year, graduates undertake the same assessment as undergraduates completing the second year of the five-year course. In the three clinical years, students are trained in the University Hospitals of Morecambe Bay and primary care centres in North Lancashire and Cumbria; the elective takes place at the end of the penultimate year. The Liverpool Medical School was ranked 22nd overall in the Complete University Guide league table.

Student review

The course

The course at Liverpool offers a one year pre-clinical phase followed by integration with the undergraduate third years for the remaining years. The Liverpool teaching style consists of a self-directed PBL system. A typical week during the first year includes a weekly self-directed session at the anatomy resource centre, four hours of supportive lectures and a half day under instruction at the clinical skills laboratory. The second, third and fourth years involve placements in large general hospitals and nationally renowned specialist hospitals where teaching and practical opportunities are varied and numerous. The unique part of the course is that, despite the focus on the medical sciences during the first year, students have very early clinical exposure, with hospital rotations starting after two months. This serves to make students both comfortable and competent in hospitals from an early stage, immediately witnessing the relevance of subjects covered in the curriculum.

The medical school/university

As a city campus, the Liverpool Medical School boasts close proximity to many hospitals and an abundance of primary care centres. In addition to the high quality of clinical experience, students benefit from modest class sizes and valuable small-group teaching in lectures and tutorials. As you would expect, the initial learning curve is steep but once the clinical years begin, students are proficient in medical sciences and a wide range of clinical skills. As well as formal teaching, there are a wide range of highly-

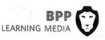

regarded societies offering additional training to students. Lectures and workshops are available on anything from general medical topics to wilderness Medicine and, not forgetting, the UK's largest student-led surgical society, the Surgical Scousers. The Liverpool Medical Students' Society is always very welcoming to graduates and boasts one of the best social calendars, from drama, debating and charity work to every type of sport. Keeping with the tradition of medics 'working hard and playing hard' mentality, Liverpool has a range of successful medics' sports teams that compete in local and national tournaments.

The local area

Liverpool is a fantastic and affordable place to live, with friendly outgoing people. In the first year, unless arranged independently, graduate students are generally placed together in halls of residence close to the university. In the remaining years students tend to move to the Smithdown Road area several miles from the university, where the majority of students live. There is great shopping available at Liverpool One and Sefton Park is a popular place to chill out in the summer. There is a great night life and something to suit most tastes, whether it be dressing up for a night out at the Albert Docks, dancing to The Beatles on Mathew Street or just sticking with the student favourite The Blue Angel, otherwise known as 'the Raz'.

Additional information

- Website address: www.liv.ac.uk/sme/prospective/graduate. htm
- Contact details:
  School of Medical Education
  MBChB Admissions Office
  Cedar House
  Ashton Street
  Liverpool
  L69 3GE

Newcastle University

- **Courses accepted**: Any degree subject.
- **Academic requirements**: A first or upper second (2:1) class Honours degree. Practising health professionals can apply with a qualification recognised by a statutory body. In addition, applicants must provide evidence of recent academic study within the last three years, such as A levels, an Open University course or GAMSAT.
- **Total intake per year**: 35
- **Applicants per place**: 25
- **Selection process**: UKCAT followed by interview.

University and course description

Newcastle University Medical School runs its courses in partnership with Durham University (at the Queen's Campus, Stockton). The pre-clinical phase occurs over the first year and is distinct from the undergraduate five-year course; teaching occurs in a problem-based 'case-led approach' in which learning objectives are drawn from clinical cases in small groups. A senior academic tutor leads and aids the group sessions and acts as an academic mentor during the first year. Clinical placements in the first year occur in both community and hospital environments. Following successful completion of the first year, graduate students follow the undergraduate course schedule. Clinical placements are widely distributed, involving the Northern Region NHS in areas such as North Cumbria, Northumbria, Tyne and Wear and Teesside. At Newcastle Medical School, the elective occurs at the end of the penultimate year. The Newcastle Medical School was ranked 8th overall in the Complete University Guide league table.

Student review

The course

The Newcastle course involves one extended pre-clinical, and three clinical, years. Accelerated students are taught separately in their first year only. The first year is mainly taught through PBL which typically takes place in two to three sessions during the week and is supervised by GP tutors. The remainder of the timetable comprises of approximately 12 hours of lectures, anatomy dissection sessions and clinical skills training. Each student is also given a patient with

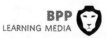
BPP
LEARNING MEDIA

a chronic illness to follow during the year and will attend a few sessions at a local GP practice. In the second year students join the undergraduate course for clinical training in one of four 'base units,' which are allocated by ballot after expressing a preference. Based within the Northern deanery, hospitals are accessible by public transport; however some students prefer to relocate. The diversity of students is one of the great advantages of the course, with graduates' subjects ranging from Music to Engineering.

The medical school/university

Located within the city centre, the medical school is attached to Newcastle's largest hospital, the Royal Victoria Infirmary. Medical school facilities are excellent and include lecture theatres, computer clusters, a medical library (with three further clusters and group learning rooms), anatomy and skills rooms, and a common room. With hospitals in Newcastle, Sunderland, Middlesbrough and Carlisle at students' disposal, most are placed on wards with only one other student, providing unparalleled learning opportunity. There are many diverse societies and causes within the university to get involved in, ranging from Inter-mural Sports to Musical Medics. There is also academic and spiritual support available to students through the university and each student is also assigned a personal tutor by the medical school at the beginning of the course. Previous years' students organise an event within the first week of term where each new student is paired with a student from the year above, who can be contacted for any queries regarding living and studying in Newcastle.

The local area

Popular areas to live in are Jesmond (with higher rental costs), Heaton and Fenham (with lower rental costs), which are all within walking distance of the medical school and have a broad spectrum of amenities without having to drive. The beauty of Newcastle is that you can be in a bustling city one moment, then strolling the beach in Tynemouth, or wandering the hills of Northumberland the next. The Metro train and bus network is cheap and convenient for getting around. Newcastle's night life is notorious nationwide, and for a good reason! There are countless bars and restaurants, as well as several theatres and cinemas (including an IMAX and Tyneside cinema for arthouse movie lovers). The city centre is home

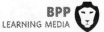

to happy hour in thrifty bars as well as the beautiful Blackfriars Restaurant, the oldest dining room in the UK. There is no shortage of activities to fill the students' free time, including the beautiful Quayside houses, the Baltic Museum and the Sage performance venue, and the Metrocentre in Gateshead – one of Europe's largest shopping centres.

Additional information
- Website address: www.ncl.ac.uk/undergraduate/course/A101
- Contact details:
  Administrator for Admissions
  Faculty Undergraduate Office
  Medical School
  Newcastle University
  Newcastle upon Tyne
  NE2 4HH
  Email (via online web form): at www.ncl.ac.uk/enquiries/

The University of Nottingham

- **Courses accepted**: Any discipline.
- **Academic requirements**: A first or upper second (2:1) class Honours degree. Masters and PhD qualifications are also accepted as an alternative to an upper second class undergraduate degree.
- **Total intake per year**: 93
- **Applicants per place**: 11
- **Selection process**: GAMSAT followed by interview using a Multiple Mini Interview (MMI) format (these occur in mid-March). Note that a minimum score of 55 in Section II, 55 in either Section I or III, and a score of at least 50 in the remaining section is required.

University and course description
The Nottingham Graduate Entry Medicine Programme is based at the Royal Derby Hospital. It involves an 18-month pre-clinical phase run separately from the undergraduate course using a predominantly PBL approach, supported by some lectures. This pre-clinical phase

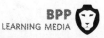

involves some early clinical exposure through GP attachments in the local area. Thereafter, the course joins the undergraduate course for a further 30 months of clinical training. These occur in placements mainly in the mid-Trent region, including hospitals in Nottinghamshire, Derbyshire, Mansfield and Lincolnshire. The elective occurs in the last nine weeks of the medical course, after the final exams. The Nottingham Medical School was ranked 27th overall in the Complete University Guide league table.

Student review

The course

The Nottingham course begins with an accelerated pre-clinical phase at the GEM school at the Royal Derby Hospital. Students then integrate with the undergraduate course for the remaining clinical phase, with placements based in large teaching hospitals and GP practices in Derbyshire, Nottinghamshire and Lincolnshire. The pre-clinical phase is divided into nine systems-based modules and focuses on PBL, supported by a series of lectures and workshops. Each week there are three PBL sessions, an Anatomy and Pathology workshop (using prosection), a clinical skills practical session and about eight hours of lectures. In addition, students spend one morning per module at a local GP surgery. Students come from a range of backgrounds: some straight out of university and others having already established successful careers. Approximately 70% of students have a Science degree, with the remaining students arriving with a variety of non science degrees – some as obscure as Egyptology!

The medical school/university

The pre-clinical phase is based in the purpose-built Medical School in Derby. It has excellent facilities including a library, lecture theatre, seminar rooms, computer clusters and around 20 PBL rooms. These rooms are well equipped with core textbooks, whiteboards, computer facilities and usually a kettle (an endless supply of tea or coffee is essential!). They become a useful base for studying and provide a safe environment to ask and discuss all those 'silly' questions. There is a strong community feel among the graduate entry students and staff, and students receive a great deal of educational and pastoral support. The base for the clinical phase is the Queen's Medical Centre in Nottingham, which is also

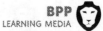

the site for the undergraduate course. Students rotate around many hospitals to maximise clinical experience. A car is therefore useful, but is not essential. Free accommodation is provided for students on placement in Mansfield and Lincoln and graduate entry students are able to claim for travel expenses.

The local area

Most graduate entry students live in Derby for the first few of years of the course. There is a variety of accommodation available including university halls of residence and private rental properties, all within a convenient walking distance of the hospital. For the final two years many students choose to relocate to Nottingham. Popular locations include Beeston, Lenton and The Park. Derby and Nottingham are both vibrant cities that boast a variety of cultural and leisure activities. There are numerous bars, clubs and restaurants and excellent shopping facilities. To escape the hustle and bustle of city life, the breathtaking Peak District is just a short drive away and features stunning landscapes. Alternatively, you can follow the Robin Hood trail through Nottingham Castle, Caves and Sherwood Forest.

Additional information

- Website address: www.nottingham.ac.uk/GEM/index.aspx
- Contact details:
  Academic Lead for Admissions
  School of Graduate Entry Medicine and Health
  Royal Derby Hospital
  Uttoxeter Road
  Derby
  DE22 3DT
  Email: gem@nottingham.ac.uk

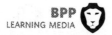

University of Oxford

- **Courses accepted**: A wide variety of scientific disciplines are accepted; an extensive list is available from the Oxford Medical School website and prospectus.
- **Academic requirements**: A first or upper second (2:1) class Honours degree. Also required are Chemistry and one other A level in a scientific subject (unless covered in a bachelors degree), together with dual-award science at GCSE level.
- **Total intake per year**: 30
- **Applicants per place**: 8
- **Selection process**: UKCAT followed by interview. In the past, candidates with an average of less than 650 per section have not been interviewed.

University and course description

Applications to Oxbridge (the collective term for the universities of Oxford and Cambridge) vary slightly from applications to other UK universities. Due to the University of Oxford being divided into colleges, an extra charge is administered, known as the 'college fee'. This is paid annually, in addition to the tuition fee, and amounts to approximately £5,000. This fee is covered by the NHS bursary in years two to four of the course, for those eligible. Candidates are able to apply to a specific college at Oxford should they wish. This provides no statistical advantage in obtaining an offer, but enables a candidate to select a preference towards a particular college as they vary significantly in terms of age, size, location and student population (some colleges admit only graduate students while others admit graduates and undergraduates). However, as teaching occurs centrally mainly, it is reasonably standardised across the colleges. It is important to note that not all colleges offer places in Graduate Medicine; for an up-to-date list, please consult the graduate course website. Unlike undergraduate applications, candidates can apply to both Oxford and Cambridge in any one year.

The first two years are spent studying with other graduate entry students only. The first year is predominantly focused on the pre-clinical material with some clinical exposure (involving weekly one day placements at GP practices and hospitals outside of Oxford), while this balance is reversed in the second year. Teaching of core topics is mostly self-directed; group sessions occur frequently and involve discussion of either clinical case research problems, or primary literature in clinical Medicine. There are few lectures on the course and students are encouraged to pursue subjects of further interest to them. In addition to group-based teaching, students are supported by weekly tutorials with a personal tutor from their college in the early years.

The final two years are integrated with the undergraduate course, and therefore it is not possible to complete the clinical years at another university (an option available to undergraduate medical students in Oxford). Clinical placements are mostly in Oxford-based hospitals, with some attachments at District General Hospitals in locations such as Milton Keynes, High Wycombe, Banbury, Stoke Mandeville, Swindon and Northampton. At Oxford, the elective takes place in the final year. Oxford Medical School was ranked 1st overall in the Complete University Guide league table.

Student review

The course

The Oxford course is very academically oriented in the pre-clinical phase. In the first year, students are expected to cover core medical knowledge on their own, and teaching hours are largely devoted to covering 'extension' topics based on research. Teaching consists of lectures and small group tutorials given through individual colleges, allowing students to personalise topic areas to be covered in tutorials. One day per week is spent on clinical attachment at a district general hospital or GP surgery. After the first year, most of the teaching is done jointly with the six-year course. Clinical training is mostly done at the Oxford Radcliffe Hospitals and surrounding District General Hospitals and GP surgeries. The course appeals to independent-types who are happy to cover large volumes of core medical knowledge on their own, and who have a keen interest in research. Of course, help is available if you struggle with core knowledge. Most students have impressive experimental Science degrees, but represent a wide range of former careers and interests.

The medical school/university

First year lectures and PBL sessions are held at the hospital and in the university's science facilities (city centre), and tutorials are

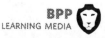

usually held in individual colleges. There is no dissection course, but anatomy sessions are held in the dissection lab to allow studying of prosections. Students tend to study in college libraries or at the hospital libraries. The John Radcliffe Hospital, the Churchill Hospital, and the Nuffield Orthopaedic Centre are the sites of many placements, and all are located a short distance outside the city centre. Most students cycle between town and these facilities. For some placements, you are required to attend local District General Hospitals, where accommodation is provided. A car is very helpful for these placements, although public transport is usually available. The graduate entry course is quite small, accepting around 30 people each year, but the undergraduate course has quite large numbers, creating an active social community.

The local area

During the first year of the course, most students live in their colleges in the city centre. In subsequent years, students tend to move out of college and find accommodation either in Headington (near to the hospitals but fewer shops and amenities) or in the Cowley area (a much more active area, but a longer cycle to the hospital).

Most students enjoy the traditions unique to Oxford, especially formal dinners in colleges, balls, spending time in Oxford's historical pubs, and punting. The strong rowing heritage means many opportunities for students to try their hand at the sport, or to enjoy life as a spectator. There is a good selection of shops, dining and nightclubs in Oxford itself, and trips into London are very easy by two bus services that schedule buses every ten minutes.

Additional information

- Website address: http://www.medsci.ox.ac.uk/study/medicine
- Contact details:
  Medical Sciences Office
  John Radcliffe Hospital
  Oxford
  OX3 9DU
  Email: enquiries@medsci.ox.ac.uk

University of Southampton

- **Courses accepted**: All subjects accepted.
- **Academic requirements**: A first or upper second (2:1) class Honours degree. A level requirements include pass at A level Chemistry or passes at AS level Biology and Chemistry. GCSEs in English, Maths and Double Science are required at grade C or above. Candidates are also expected to show evidence of recent study.
- **Total intake per year**: 40
- **Applicants per place**: 36
- **Selection process**: UKCAT; there is no interview for admission.

University and course description

The Graduate Entry Medicine course at Southampton has a less defined division between clinical and pre-clinical Medicine than many other courses. While the final two years of the course are primarily clinical and assimilated with the undergraduate course, the first two years involve learning a mixture of basic science and clinical Medicine. Some lectures are held conjointly with those from the five-year course. The style of learning is principally PBL (with some additional lectures) in which students work in groups with a facilitator. The first two years consist of four semesters (totalling 30 weeks) and a curriculum using clinical topics as a framework for learning. Clinical exposure is both community and hospital based in the first two years, typically involving two or three clinical sessions each week. Hospital clinical work takes place at the Royal Hampshire County Hospital, Winchester. Years three and four are identical to the principal course. The elective takes place in the penultimate year. Southampton Medical School was ranked 29th overall in the Complete University Guide league table.

Student review

The course

The first two years of the course at Southampton is centred on clinical topics which form the basis for each week's learning. This takes place as a combination of PBL-type discussions, lectures, anatomy practical sessions and clinical teaching. Supplementary to this, students are expected to undertake self-directed learning to fulfil

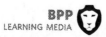

the rest of the learning outcomes. Each week culminates in a plenary session with an expert in that particular field of Medicine. Clinical teaching in the first two years is based at Winchester Hospital (every week) and through primary care attachments (every other week). At the end of each year students are examined on their clinical skills by an observed structured clinical examination. Students join their five-year colleagues in their third and fourth year where clinical attachments are the mainstay of the programme. The course ensures that any student has the potential to succeed regardless of their individual background and as such Southampton accept applications from students with degrees in any discipline.

The medical school/university

Although the medical school is based at Southampton General Hospital (SGH), teaching on the course takes place across three main sites: SGH, Winchester Royal Hampshire County Hospital and the main Highfield campus, which saw the opening of a new fifty million pound Life Sciences building in 2011. As expected from a leading research university, facilities are excellent throughout all three main teaching sites. SGH boasts its own health services library and a dedicated 'Centre for Learning Anatomical Sciences' which itself has recently been refurbished, offering various prosected specimens for teaching sessions. There is a large number of sports clubs and societies associated with the medical school which ensure students are always kept busy. Pastoral support throughout the course is excellent and this is aided in part by a student mentoring scheme beginning in the first year.

The local area

With a student population of around 30,000, accommodation is certainly not difficult to find in Southampton – there is the option of a place in halls of residence for first-year students, while in the following years students tend to live in shared houses in either the Highfield or Portswood areas, or near the SGH. As the course has a fairly small intake each cohort tends to form a close-knit group, both academically and socially. Nightlife in Southampton is quite varied – if the desire is to relive previous student days then that is more than catered for by pubs and clubs in Portswood; however for a more refined night out Bedford Place is slightly more upmarket with some fairly classy establishments. Other attractions include

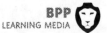

some of the best comprising of shopping facilities on the South coast and Southampton Common – 326 acres of parkland next to the campus.

Additional information

- Website address: www.som.soton.ac.uk/undergrad/course/bm4
- Contact details:
  School of Medicine Admissions Office
  Southampton General Hospital
  Tremona Road
  Southampton
  Hampshire
  SO16 6YD
  Email: bmadmissions@southampton.ac.uk

St George's, University of London

- **Courses accepted**: Any degree discipline.
- **Academic requirements**: Minimum of a lower second (2:2) class Honours degree. Masters and PhD qualifications are accepted as an alternative.
- **Total intake per year**: 98
- **Applicants per place**: 9
- **Selection process**: GAMSAT followed by MMI, which involves seven stations which applicants rotate around. Examples of these are available on the St George's website. Interviews are held in January. Each year, St George's sets a minimum overall GAMSAT score that is published on its website. Candidates must also achieve a score of at least 55 in Section II, 55 in either Section I or III, and 50 in the remaining section to be considered for interview.

University and course description

The St George's graduate course began in 2000 and is the longest established in the UK. The pre-clinical teaching at St George's lasts one year and follows a PBL structure where different medical scenarios or case histories are explored with a tutor each week. Clinical experience occurs from the outset in various hospital and

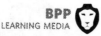

community settings. The majority of the basic science teaching takes place at the main Tooting site, which is approximately 20 minutes from central London, while up to two-thirds of clinical training occurs at different sites. The final three years are integrated with the five-year course. The second year is designed to act as a transitional year between pre-clinical and clinical Medicine, with the final two years concentrating primarily on clinical Medicine. The elective is undertaken in the final year. St George's Medical School was ranked 23rd overall in the Complete University Guide league table.

Student review

The course

From day one, there is a huge emphasis on clinical experience and practice, with a large portion of the science based studies being self-directed, which requires students to be independent and confident, supported by lectures on underlying principles. The second year, known as the 'transitional' year sees students merge with the undergraduate students into a 50:50 mix of clinical placements and PBL sessions. The final two years give students a broad experience across almost every specialty, with several SSCs providing the opportunity to study or practise in a specific area of interest beyond the syllabus. There is a huge emphasis on integration, not just with undergraduates but with all healthcare programmes at the medical school, which is the last standalone medical college in the country. Clinical placements are varied, and though there are occasional distant placements for which accommodation is provided, this is never more than twice a year and balanced so that no student receives more than others. Case-based discussions with mini-clinical examinations means that students are encouraged to engage with and get the most from their placements.

The medical school/university

The current site in Tooting is situated with St George's NHS Trust Hospital, one of the busiest in Europe. Student accommodation is within walking distance of the medical school, saving money on travelling. St George's considers itself the friendliest Medical School in the land, and never fails to deliver. It is a small family of healthcare professionals, where you can walk out of a lecture or the wards into the onsite SU bar and enjoy a pint with your peers, lecturers, doctors and nurses alike. Teaching facilities are brand new and still expanding, and there is always rapid response to student demand. The only downside is that the size inevitably means that facilities do sometimes reach capacity, especially during exams. St George's offers much pastoral care, along with plenty of societies, from the art societies who put on shows, to volunteer societies. St George's is heavily involved in charity work – and sports teams with a sports centre hosting every sport you could want.

The local area

You are never short of a curry house in Tooting! It is a vibrant and multicultural environment. While it is very cheap as far as London goes, it is also seeing rapid development, already unrecognisable from five years ago. High street stores are replacing the numerous poundshops, along with pubs and swanky bars, catering more to the young professional than the local lager lout. The hospital itself is next to Tooting Broadway and you are a short Northern Line ride away from central London (20 minutes away) along with numerous busy bus routes and overground stations. There are also two night buses into central London, though many students do not feel the need to venture far, as the union bar within the hospital is a hub of student activity, events and parties. Nearby there is a nature centre, Wandsworth Common for walks in the park, a leisure centre, an ice rink, golf course, horse-riding, the largest open-air swimming pool in the UK, rowing at Chiswick on the Thames and sailing at Royal Victoria Dock and greyhound racing at Wimbledon stadium.

Additional information

- Website address: www.sgul.ac.uk/courses undergraduate
- Contact details:
  Medical Admissions Officer
  St George's University of London
  Cranmer Terrace
  London
  SW17 0RE
  Email: enquiries@sgul.ac.uk

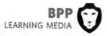

Swansea University

- **Courses accepted**: Any degree discipline.
- **Academic requirements**: A first or upper second (2:1) class Honours degree. An AS or A level in a Biology or Chemistry is preferred. A grade C in Maths is the minimum required at GSCE level.
- **Total intake per year**: 70
- **Applicants per place**: 10
- **Selection process**: GAMSAT followed by interview.

University and course description

Launched in 2004, the medical programme at Swansea University is one of only two courses that caters solely for graduate students (the other being the University of Warwick); there is no undergraduate five-year course. The first two years of the course are mainly campus-based, exploring a clinical problem through group tutorials, lectures and seminars. Some of the course is taught through a PBL approach. Clinical attachments to hospitals take place in the final two years, involving the Abertawe Bro Morgannwg University Health Board, and are based entirely in Swansea and the West Wales area. The elective takes place in the penultimate year. Swansea Medical School was not ranked in the last Complete University Guide league table.

Student review

The course

The Swansea course is considered fairly innovative with a two-year case-based taught programme followed by a two-year clinical phase. The case-based element of the course covers all the various elements of Medicine and includes three clinical placements. The week begins with a clinical case presentation followed by various lectures, using a spiral learning model (which covers the fundamentals then returns to them in more detail later). In addition there are half-day clinical skills each week, monthly visits to a local GP surgery and three five-week hospital placements. The second phase of the programme is currently in evolution as students in previous years have moved to Cardiff University to complete their degree. It is envisaged that the final two years will be in Swansea and West Wales and will involve 13 clinical placements,

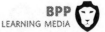

an elective period in year three and a shadowing period at the end of year four.

The medical school/university

Swansea Medical School is located in the former Chemistry building of Swansea University and has a small anatomy suite (with models and prosections), a computer suite and a clinical skills lab. As a very small medical school, the resources available are adequate for the small cohort. Most teaching takes place in lecture theatres and dedicated teaching rooms. Although all teaching takes place on campus, it is advantageous to have a car while studying in Swansea – only Singleton Hospital is close to the town centre, all others are a fair distance and public transport is not recommended other than to Morrison Hospital. GP surgeries can be located over 50 miles away in the Welsh countryside. Swansea University is officially the closest university to the sea in the world, with only a main road separating the main leafy campus to the beach. The university itself is located in Singleton Park with a pretty boating lake, playing fields and outstanding views of the bay.

The local area

Swansea University is around two miles from the town centre on the seafront and the majority of students live within a 15-minute walk of the university in Brynmill or Uplands. Uplands has a village feel and includes popular pubs, shops and eateries. Swansea town centre has a good selection of shops, although Cardiff is 50 minutes on the train for more serious shopping. There are regular bus services from the university and student areas to the town centre and central railway station. Swansea is a medium-sized town so the nightlife varies. The majority of pubs and bars can be located in Wind Street which is a bustling hive of activity at weekends and there are regular student nights in the week. The marina area has a small range of more upmarket restaurants and bars. By far, Swansea's biggest draw is the fantastic coastal and country scenery on offer. Nearby Gower is an area of outstanding natural beauty and is a haven for watersports fans and walkers alike.

Additional information

- Website address: www.swan.ac.uk/ugcourses/medicine/ mbbchmedicinegraduateentry/
- Contact details:
  Swansea University
  College of Medicine
  Graduate Entry Programme
  Swansea
  SA2 8PP
  Email: medicine@swansea.ac.uk

University of Warwick

- **Courses accepted**: Courses in biological, health, natural or physical sciences. See the Warwick Medical School website for a complete list of accepted degree titles.
- **Academic requirements:** A first or upper second (2:1) class Honours degree, though applicants with a lower second (2:2) may be considered if they have attained a PhD qualification.
- **Total intake per year**: 178
- **Applicants per place**: 9
- **Selection process**: UKCAT followed by an assessment centre based interview.

University and course description

As well as having the largest Graduate Medicine Programme in the UK, Warwick Medical School is one of only two universities (along with Swansea University) to run a four-year programme with no parallel five-year undergraduate course. The course has been running since 2000 and is divided into two phases. The first phase lasts 18 months and takes place over three semesters. Teaching mainly occurs on campus, with early clinical placements at University Hospitals in Coventry and Warwickshire and primary care placements in the surrounding areas. In this first phase, students are taught mainly via lectures and small learning groups, guided by facilitators who are either clinicians or academic members of staff. Groups are formed specifically to include students from a range of different ages and backgrounds. The second phase concentrates on clinical Medicine and takes place in 12 eight-week clinical blocks in hospitals located in Coventry, Nuneaton, Redditch, Rugby and Warwick. The elective takes place in the penultimate year. Warwick Medical School was ranked 14th overall in the Complete University Guide league table.

Student review

The course

The course at Warwick is made up of one and a half years of 'phase one' which covers the bulk of the teaching, and two and half years of 'phase two' which includes placements in and around Coventry and Warwickshire, and a six-week elective period. Phase one is primarily based on campus and consists of lectures and small group sessions to reinforce the learning as well the use of plastinated models to visualise anatomical teaching. There is also a one day/afternoon clinical placement per week in the community, or on hospital wards which are used to get early patient exposure and to build on history taking and clinical skills. From the outset, students are taught not only the science but the clinical application and practice of the skills required in Medicine. Medical students at Warwick come from a range of backgrounds including non-scientific degrees and careers, creating a diverse cohort with a range of skill sets.

The medical school/university

The University of Warwick campus is situated over 290 hectares of land on the outskirts of Coventry and contains much greenery including lakes and woods. It offers extensive, affordable sports facilities and excellent teaching facilities. The Medical Teaching Centre (MTC) was opened in 2000, and has very modern facilities including a main lecture theatre, small group rooms, a computer room and students common room. Students have access to a range of anatomical models, books and examination rooms and equipment within the MTC and the biomedical sciences library, situated next to the MTC. Prosection teaching is done at the new Surgical Training Centre at University Hospital, Coventry and Warwickshire, and the opportunity to take part in dissection is available during the summer, after the first year.

The local area

During the first year of the course, a few students live in halls on campus, however the majority live in Coventry, Kenilworth, Leamington Spa or further afield. Most students eventually live in Leamington Spa, a beautiful town which does not conform to the traditional 'student' image, so is ideally suited for postgraduate living. The campus itself, and Coventry, Kenilworth and Leamington Spa have all of the services and amenities you could desire, including great restaurants, pubs and cafes – ranging from the traditional to the modern. Nightlife is varied, from large clubs in Coventry and the Student Union, to smaller clubs and pubs in Leamington Spa; with the occasional trip further afield (such as Birmingham, which is not too far away). In additional to normal club nights, there are regular and varied events organised by the Medical Society and medics sports teams that are always popular.

Additional information

* Website address: www2.warwick.ac.uk/fac/med/study/ugr/
* Contact details:
  Admissions Office
  Warwick Medical School
  The University of Warwick
  Coventry
  CV4 7AL
  Email (via online contact form): www2.warwick.ac.uk/study/postgraduate/contacts/pgenquiry

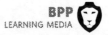

Summary

- The profiles above of the UK medical schools offering graduate entry courses are designed to help you in selecting courses for your application.
- Remember that students' experiences will vary greatly within any particular course, so as well as reading the student reviews in this chapter, try to speak to as many students as you can at the medical schools you are considering applying to.
- Aim to attend the open days run by the medical schools as these are excellent sources of information.
- For those wishing to consult detailed and objective comparisons of the performance of the different Medicine courses, the reports of the GMC's assessments of each school are available from their website.

 ## Useful resources

www.thecompleteuniversityguide.co.uk
www.medschoolsonline.co.uk
www.gmc-uk.org

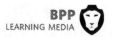

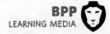

Chapter 5

The UCAS application and personal statement

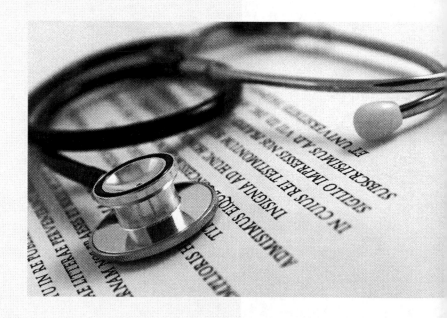

Chapter 5

The UCAS application and personal statement

The UCAS form is the first piece of information that Medical Schools receive about an applicant and, along with your entrance exam results, is the major determinant of whether you will be short-listed for interview. A key part of the UCAS form is the personal statement, a section that instills fear in many applicants due to the significance attributed to it by many medical schools when inviting candidates for interview. Given this importance, it is paramount that it be written to the highest possible standard. The first half of the chapter reviews each section of the UCAS form, including the information you will need in order to complete it. The second half of the chapter will discuss the personal statement in more detail, offering advice on how to structure your own personal statement and what to include to impress the admissions panel.

When to apply

Applications for Medicine courses (both undergraduate and graduate entry) open in mid-September for admission in the following September or October. Please check the UCAS website for details of opening and closing dates for the particular year in which you apply. Provided your application arrives by the application deadline, you should not be disadvantaged, however, UCAS sends batches of applications to universities in the order that they arrive, and some universities make offers on a continuous basis, therefore your application should be sent in a timely manner. Only one UCAS application can be submitted per year and up to four medical schools may be included in any one application.

How to apply

Application to all Graduate Entry Medicine courses is made online via the UCAS website. When registering for the first time you will be asked whether you are applying through an institution. As a graduate, it is likely that you will classify as an independent student, which allows you to apply without the involvement of your former school, or college. Following registration, your profile can be saved each time you access your account, allowing you to complete the form in multiple sittings. If you anticipate not being able to access your UCAS account for a period of time, in the first part of the online form there is the opportunity to nominate another individual to gain access to your account, and to make decisions on your behalf.

There are six sections on the UCAS form which fall under the headings: personal details, choices, education, employment, personal statement and references. To complete your application as an independent student, you will need the following information:

- Personal details, including permanent home address, fee code status and, if applicable, reference numbers for the International English Language Testing System (IELTS) or Test of English as a Foreign Language (TOEFL).
- Passport details (if a non EU student).
- Your choices of university or universities, and course codes (Graduate Entry Medicine is usually A101, however, at King's College London, the code is A102).
- Details of all schools and colleges you have attended since the age of eleven.
- Details of all relevant qualifications which have been awarded, or are ongoing. You will also need the examination centre number for schools and colleges where you have sat exams. (This can be searched for automatically during the UCAS application procedure.)
- Details of paid employment.
- Personal statement.
- Reference statement.
- A Visa, Mastercard, Maestro or Solo card to pay the application fee. The fee is £11 if you are applying to one course and £22 if you are applying to two or more courses.

Personal details

In the personal details section of the application, you are required to enter a valid email address – be aware that this address will be visible to the medical schools you apply to, so ensure it is suitably professional. You will also be asked to supply details of your fee code, which will depend on your student status. Students from the following countries are normally classified as 'home' students: England, Scotland, Wales, Northern Ireland, The Channel Islands, The Isle of Man and students from the European Union (EU), which

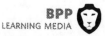

has a fee code of 02. Students from outside these regions, including students from the USA, Canada, Australia and New Zealand, are normally classified as 'overseas' students, which has a fee code of 01. A number of other fee code options exist for students receiving funding from alternative sources. If you are unsure of your fee code, or the residency criteria for 'home' status, consult the website of the UK Council for International Student Affairs (www.ukcisa.org. uk). The personal details section also requests details on English proficiency and any criminal convictions.

Choices

You are allowed to apply to a maximum of four medical courses, which may be all graduate entry, all undergraduate or a mixture of the two courses. UCAS arranges your choices alphabetically and not in order of preference. Furthermore, each university will not see details of any other courses to which you have applied. Note that Oxford and Cambridge University courses require a further form to be completed in addition to the UCAS form. Details of these application forms are available at the respective course website.

Education

To complete the education section of the application form, you will need the details of all your educational qualifications to date. In addition to this, you are also required to state:

- Courses you have been enrolled on (even if you have since withdrawn from the course, or still have exams to complete).
- Courses which you are awaiting the results of.
- Courses which you received an unsuccessful grade or are re-sitting.

For A level or AS level courses you will also have the option of listing the grades you have achieved for each module. For instructions on entering other qualifications, including Scottish Highers, the Welsh Baccalaureate and the Irish Leaving Certificate please refer to the UCAS website. It is not necessary to send university transcripts with your UCAS form, although it is a good idea to start requesting them, as they may be required by a university at a later date. Results of admission tests, such as the GAMSAT, BMAT and UKCAT can be inserted under 'Additional Admissions Tests', however, these results are also supplied to universities directly and therefore it is not mandatory to include them on the UCAS form.

Employment

Details of up to five employers can be entered in the employment section. UCAS recommends that details of unpaid work experience are entered in the personal statement section, rather than the employment section. Once the application has been processed by UCAS, details of additional employment can be sent directly to universities and colleges, if you feel that this would benefit your application.

References

Prior to submitting the UCAS form, one reference will be required in full. As an independent applicant, it is your personal responsibility to submit the reference supplied by your referee. UCAS do not permit references from family, friends, partners or ex-partners and may cancel your application if this is found to be the case. Suitable people to ask for a reference may be a personal tutor at university or another member of the academic staff who is familiar with your work. Alternatively, you may want to ask a clinician you have worked with or shadowed. Suggested topics you may ask your referee to comment on include:

- Commitment to Medicine.
- Academic ability and potential.
- Academic interests.
- Attributes required for Medicine, such as communication skills, empathy, honesty, integrity, and propensity for teamwork.
- Mitigating circumstances (please note: health related issues can only be included with your permission).
- Areas not covered in your personal statement.

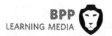

Further notes for applicants

Applicants to Oxford and Cambridge

Unlike at undergraduate level, applicants to Graduate Entry Medicine are permitted to apply to both the Universities of Oxford and Cambridge. Both courses require the completion of a separate application form, in addition to the UCAS application form, which are available from their respective websites. The University of Oxford requires three references, and the University of Cambridge requires two references to accompany the application. Oxford Medical School requires applicants to sit the UKCAT test before an application is submitted, while applicants to Cambridge may sit the BMAT if they do not meet the pre-medical requirements. An additional fee of £15 is charged for applications to Cambridge.

International students

Students from outside the UK should apply via UCAS in the same way as UK students. If you are an applicant from outside the European Union (EU) or European Economic Area (EEA), the number of four-year courses which you can apply to is limited. At present, the following medical schools will consider such applications: the University of Warwick, Imperial College London, King's College London, The University of Nottingham, the University of Oxford and the University of Southampton.

Students from within the EU, EEA or Swiss Nationals are normally eligible to apply to courses in the same way as UK students, however a small number of medical schools (such as the University of Bristol) will only accept degrees completed in the UK. Therefore, if you have completed your degree outside the UK, you are strongly advised to contact your preferred medical schools early in the process to gain clarification on your eligibility.

Universities have varying policies on language requirements for applicants whose first language is not English, and information is usually provided on the medical school website. A typical requirement is an International English Language Testing System (IELTS) score of 7, or a Test of English as a Foreign Language (TOEFL) score of 100, with minimum scores in particular sections. Please note that EU students will not normally be eligible for an

NHS bursary during years two to four of the course and will therefore be required to pay full tuition fees each year.

Deferred entry

The option of deferred entry is generally not encouraged for four-year courses, and a number of medical schools will not consider deferred applications at all. One exception is King's College London, which does permit applications for deferred entry. In exceptional circumstances, other medical schools may permit deferred entry once a place has been secured on a course. Any conditions attached to an offer for deferred entry must be met in the same year as the application is submitted, usually by 31st August, which means that it is not normally possible to use the time spent during a deferred year to meet the entry requirements specified in the conditional offer.

Criminal records

All UK applicants to medical school will undergo an enhanced criminal records bureau (CRB) check, which will reveal current and spent convictions, cautions and reprimands held on the Police National Computer, as well as any relevant information held by local police forces. Checks of the Children and Vulnerable Adults barred lists can also be made at this time. International applicants are asked to undertake an equivalent check in their home country prior to entry into the UK.

Criminal offences should be declared along with the UCAS application; full details should also be sent to the medical schools to which you are applying. The GMC advise that all convictions, no matter how old, should be declared. It is not necessary to supply evidence of any road traffic offences where you have accepted the option of paying a fixed penalty notice.

Occupational health

An occupational health screening questionnaire may be sent out prior to starting medical school. Medical students are likely to be screened for immunity against (or infection of) Hepatitis B, tuberculosis, rubella, measles, mumps and varicella. Some medical schools require a completed course of Hepatitis B immunisations

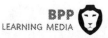

before admission, and it is important to note that this course may take up to six months to complete. Under the Department of Health guidance, students with blood borne viruses are not automatically excluded from studying Medicine, and students are advised to contact the respective medical school early in the process for advice about this, or any other occupational health issues.

What happens after you apply?

Following submission of your application, you will receive a letter confirming your choice of universities. Each university will then individually assess your application in order to decide whether to invite you to interview. You can track the progress of your application on the UCAS Track website (www.ucas.ac.uk/students/ track). UCAS requires all universities to make decisions by the end of March, however for popular courses such as Medicine, final decisions may not be made until early May. Should you receive a conditional offer, you must meet the conditions of the offer by the deadline, which is usually the end of August. Some conditions may have to be met earlier, particularly if you are taking exams during winter.

Replying to offers

When all of your chosen universities have arrived at a decision, you will be required to reply to all offers by a certain deadline, which will vary depending on the date that the last university made their decision. It is vital that you reply to all offers by this date, or your offers will be automatically declined on your behalf by UCAS. If you have received multiple offers, you are able to accept one offer as a firm acceptance and a second as an insurance choice. The insurance choice can be either conditional or unconditional. However, if your first choice is unconditional, you will not be able to select an insurance choice. It is important to note that it is highly unlikely that a Graduate Entry Medicine course will be available via UCAS clearing or UCAS Extra.

The personal statement

The personal statement is a significant aspect of any UCAS application and, along with your academic and entrance exam results, determines whether a medical school will offer you an

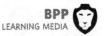

interview. As most applicants to Graduate Entry Medicine will have a similarly strong academic record, the personal statement provides an opportunity to distinguish yourself from other applicants by conveying your own individual story. The personal statement is also important once you have been short listed for interview, as it often forms the basis of several questions. This is one reason why it is important to be completely honest with your application as if you have been found to have embellished your personal statement at interview, your application to that medical school, and possibly others, will be over.

Before exploring the personal statement in detail, there are a few practicalities worth noting. As with all sections of the UCAS application, the personal statement is completed online. You are able to enter up to 4,000 characters for your personal statement (which includes spaces), or 47 lines of text. As there is no spelling or grammar check function on the UCAS website, it is advisable to write the statement in a word processing program and then copy and paste it into the online form. Avoid the use of complex formatting, such as variable font sizes, as this will be lost when pasted onto the form.

There are many ways to write a personal statement and indeed, many things that could be included. It is essential that you give due consideration to both the form and content of your personal statement; as it should be engaging and memorable, yet also feature certain key pieces of information expected by Admissions Officers. A number of excerpts from personal statements are used for illustrative purposes below, however you are reminded that these are examples to use as a guide when writing your own personal statement and should not be copied directly.

For many, the most difficult part of writing the personal statement is creating an initial draft. The first thing to decide upon is what information to include. It can also be helpful at this stage to consider the structure of your personal statement, which you can then subsequently add detail to. Below is an example of a basic structure you could consider:

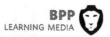

Paragraph 1:	Begin with a memorable opening statement and a brief explanation of why you want to study Medicine.
Paragraphs 2 and 3:	Give an account of the work and voluntary experience you have acquired to gain an insight into the field of Medicine. For each key experience, outline what you have learned from it. As a final point, mention which areas of Medicine and Surgery you are particularly interested in.
Paragraph 4:	Incorporate any information that does not fit conveniently into the other paragraphs, for example, you could include research experience, or significant life experiences related to Medicine. You could also give an account of your academic background in this paragraph.
Paragraph 5:	In the final paragraph briefly discuss your extra-curricular activities. Finally, close with a statement to reiterate your suitability towards Medicine.

Introduction

The obvious starting point is to explain why you want to study Medicine. It is your opportunity to gain the reader's attention and interest so it is important that it makes an impression. The answer to this question can often be clichéd, therefore it is best to avoid the ubiquitous 'I like Science and want to help people' as this will have little impact on the admissions tutors. Admittedly, these may be your main motivations, however, for an application to stand out, this must be presented in a novel or interesting way.

A good starting point is to consider what is unique about you, or your life experiences. Explain how and when you became interested in Medicine; perhaps there have been personal or family illnesses, or influential individuals who have inspired you and shaped your career aspirations. Your suitability towards Medicine will appear more convincing if you present your points using solid and specific experiences. It is best to avoid statements why you did not originally study Medicine upon leaving school or college, and instead, concentrate on your present motivations. The following is an example of a good opening statement:

> *A medical degree will enable me to achieve my ambition of pursuing a stimulating and challenging career, through which I can make a genuine contribution to the well being of others. A range of work experiences have given me a realistic expectation of the demands placed upon a doctor and confirmed my enjoyment of working with healthcare professionals and patients.*

A similarly impressive, but slightly different approach is:

> *My personal desire to follow Medicine as a career has been sharpened through my experience over the past five years of family members with Parkinson's disease, cancers, stroke and orthopaedic trauma.*

Once you have explained why you wish to study Medicine, your introduction should then demonstrate that you have adequately researched the career, and gained insight into the world of Medicine. This is your opportunity to display the efforts you have made to learn about the profession, through any of a number of ways, including voluntary or paid work, personal experiences, or discussions with medical students and doctors. Discussing your experience serves two purposes: it highlights your interest in Medicine, and also reassures the medical school that you have not entered into a medical career lightly.

Work experience

As Medicine is a vocational career, it is essential that you include in your personal statement supporting evidence that you actually want to work with people who are unwell, therefore this section of the personal statement is particularly significant. A common mistake by applicants, particularly to Graduate Entry Medicine, is to place too much emphasis on academic credentials at the expense of their clinical experience. Therefore, although you will undoubtedly have many impressive academic achievements you could include, you should focus on your clinical experience related to Medicine.

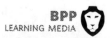

When outlining your work experience it is important to include sufficient detail to give the reader a true impression of your experience. Information you may want to include is: the name of the hospital (or healthcare setting) you were based at, the period of time you were there, and the responsibilities and activities you were involved in. Also, when describing your work experience it is best to avoid generalities, such as:

> From my work experience I have seen that Medicine offers the challenges and teamwork I am looking for in a career.

Although this sentence may be accurate, it is somewhat uninspiring, and tells the reader very little about the applicant. You must attempt to show the reader that you have actually experienced or observed these challenges personally. The key to avoiding generalisation and clichés is to imbed your statements with real world examples. Contrast the above experience to the following student's account of volunteering as a hospital attendant:

> I helped invalid patients eat, delivered samples to the laboratories and took patients to radiology and surgery [...] I had the opportunity to interact with the entire hospital staff from cleaner to consultant, and from patients with minor ailments to those who were terminally ill.

Furthermore, when recounting your experiences of Medicine, ensure any medical terminology you use is accurately and appropriately employed. Another common mistake that may befall applicants is listing numerous experiences at the expense of describing what they gained from the experience. Medical schools are more interested in how a particular experience has shaped your conviction to study medicine, rather than a long list of placements lacking detail. You should convey to the reader that you like people and find them interesting and not that you perceive Medicine in the context of intellectualism.

You should also explain how your experience has influenced your personal development and what you have learnt about yourself, as this ability to introspect is highly regarded by medical schools. The following excerpt is a good example of what a student learnt from their experience, and what they learned about their self:

I was able to develop my communication skills during conversations with patients, and I found this opportunity aided my understanding by actively listening to them. I realised that I find talking to patients extremely gratifying as it enables me to see the positive effects I could have in improving their health and wellbeing. This experience also impressed upon me the importance of sensitive and empathic communication skills, which helps establish a trusting relationship between doctor and patient.

Presenting your experience in this manner, allied with a genuine sense of enthusiasm, should confer an advantage over other applicants.

Other information

At this stage of the statement you may wish to detail any personal hardships or obstacles you have encountered, such as health related problems. The following is an example of how a student developed a particular clinical interest through a personal experience:

Although I am entirely open to all areas of Medicine, I have a deep and personal interest in oncology. I spent eight weeks with my brother who needed chemo and radiotherapy for nasopharyngeal cancer in 2006. I really admired the clinical expertise of the oncologist, and was equally inspired by his adaptive communication skill and carefully judged sense of optimism.

This type of statement could enhance your application, as it is another example of a valuable learning experience and strength of character, which could serve you well as a future doctor. It may also be worthwhile to include your career aspirations if you have thought about than, as a career plan suggests you have considered your future beyond medical school.

In this paragraph you could also include any information that does not fit suitably elsewhere, for example, you could mention your academic or research experience, but be careful not to give too much detail, as some of this information can be included in other parts of the UCAS form, such as the section on previous employment.

Extra-curricular activities

Finally, a good personal statement should include a paragraph on your personal characteristics, skills and other interests. The key objective throughout the personal statement is to convey to the admissions officer that you are the most suitable candidate for a place on their course. Essentially, your aim is to demonstrate that you possess the perceived characteristics of a good doctor, outlined in *Tomorrow's Doctors* (2009) which includes being considerate, trustworthy and acting with integrity. One way to display that you possess these qualities is through your work and outside interests, as shown in this excellent example:

> *Through my role as co-founder of the MEDSIN branch at St. Andrews University [...] I was responsible for recruitment of a number of speakers from around the UK to lecture on healthcare provision in developing societies [...] also involved medical students in the teaching of basic life support in local schools, a role which required recruitment, training and allocation of volunteers, as well as initial liaison with school co-ordinators.*

In this section, you should emphasise your involvement in teams and highlight responsibilities you have held, for example through sports clubs, societies, volunteer organisations and professional experiences. You must present yourself as a well-rounded individual that participates in a variety of extra-curricular activities. A poor example of a well-rounded individual is:

> *In my spare time I enjoy socialising with my friends by going to the pub.*

The aim is to demonstrate that you use your free time effectively. This expectation may be higher for graduate applicants than for school leavers. You should concisely mention hobbies not directly related to Medicine, such as reading, music or sport, as this displays your ability to manage your time to include relaxation, and displays that you are a balanced person. Contrast the previous example with this superior account of sport participation:

> *As an enthusiastic runner, I have chaired the University Athletics Club and volunteered at international Cerebral Palsy athletics events. Furthermore, through coaching and mentoring young athletes I have gained immense personal satisfaction.*

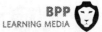

Again, remember to be specific; for example, if you mention reading then name an author that has particularly inspired you. Finally, ensure that you can elaborate on everything you mention in your personal statement, as at the interview, you may be asked to expand on it.

Concluding statement and final checks

As is the case with every piece of writing, you need a summary in which you can reiterate how important it is to you to be offered the opportunity to study Medicine. You should briefly restate your desire to pursue Medicine, having undergone a period of reflection and deliberation, and remind the reader of the qualities you possess to make you particularly suitable to becoming a doctor. The following is an example of a strong closing statement:

> *After much balanced thought, I am confident that my tenacity, stamina and wider experience will enable me to cope with these aspects of medical practice and the considerable amount of training over the next decade.*

The language throughout your personal statement should be clear and simple. Two key elements worth incorporating into your statement are an appropriate enthusiasm for the subject and a quiet confidence; acknowledge that you are an impressive candidate but be careful not to verge on arrogance! Finally, it is of paramount importance to check your statement once completed for spelling, grammar and punctuation. Try to find alternative ways of starting sentences other than 'I', and similarly, ensure that you have not repeated words, or included long, unfocused sentences. Remember that it creates a very poor impression if there are mistakes, as one would not expect carelessness from a future medical student.

Summary

- There are many ways that you can impress the reader in your personal statement, and the advice given in this chapter is by no means exhaustive.
- Your personal statement is your story, and you should try to convey this to the reader using your own personal experiences, whilst doing your utmost to avoid generalities.
- A golden rule is to avoid boring your reader, so endeavour to keep your statement interesting, and where possible, distinct.
- Allowing yourself sufficient time to reflect upon your personal experiences, which have lead you to arrive at your decision to become a doctor, will allow you to write with authority and impressive conviction.

 Useful resource

www.ucas.ac.uk/students/apply

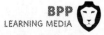

Chapter 6

Work experience and extra-curricular activities

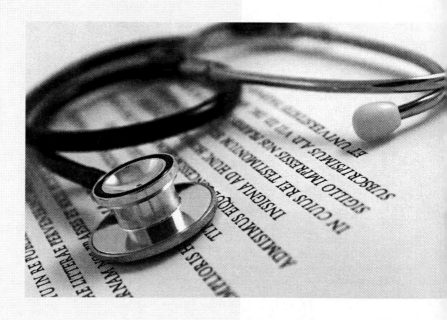

Work experience and extra-curricular activities

Work experience is a vital aspect of applying to medical school, as it fulfils two major objectives. First, gaining work experience helps prospective medical students to decide whether a career in Medicine is right for them, and second, evidence of work experience is an essential requirement of every Graduate Entry Medicine course. This chapter discusses reasons why work experience is vital to your application and the types of work experience which will enable you to gain the most valuable experiences. The chapter also considers the importance of extra-curricular activities in the assessment process.

Why is work experience important?

Receiving an offer to medical school not only means securing a place on the course, but also represents the first step towards entering the medical profession. Therefore, an important task faced by medical schools is identifying the applicants most suited to become future doctors. A career in Medicine requires a strong work ethic, a caring nature and the highest standards of professionalism as reflected in *Tomorrow's Doctors* (2009) and a well planned work experience placement can demonstrate all of these qualities. One of the key areas that interviewers are concerned with is ensuring that applicants have a realistic expectation of the role of a doctor. It is therefore essential that you have worked, or volunteered in a healthcare setting to ensure you are familiar with the environment you will be spending a large part of your professional life in. A carefully considered work experience placement will demonstrate that you fully understand what a career in Medicine entails – not just what you have seen on the television!

As well as being an essential part of the application process, work experience and volunteering provides many other benefits. Many applicants find it an enjoyable and informative experience, helping to confirm their intention to pursue a medical career. Furthermore, investing time and energy back into the wider community can be an extremely rewarding experience and by learning to balance work experience with your other commitments you will be able to develop your skills in time management.

All medical schools expect some form of work experience to have been undertaken, and some specify a minimum amount of work experience they expect candidates to possess. You should therefore consult with the medical schools you are interested in applying to at an early stage to ensure you are able to meet any work experience requirements. If you are offered an interview you can expect to be questioned on your previous work experience, therefore, you should prepare for questions about your work experience (see Chapter 8 for more information regarding the medical school interview). An additional advantage of gaining work experience is that you will start to develop an awareness of current medical issues which will further inform your answers during the interview.

It is important to recognise that as well as ensuring you have gained work experience of sufficient length, it should also enable you to gain valuable clinical experience. Spending time in a variety of healthcare settings is an effective way to gain an appreciation of the breadth of Medicine. The daily activities of a Surgeon, a Psychiatrist and a General Practitioner will differ greatly and spending time with these doctors will yield very diverse, yet equally worthwhile experience. Attempting to combine breadth and depth to your work experience will not only strengthen your insight into Medicine, but also carries the additional benefit of helping to distinguish you from other applicants. It is therefore advisable, in the course of submitting your application that you maximise every opportunity to gain varied work experience. This will broaden your clinical experience and also demonstrate your determination to learn more about the environments doctors work in.

Essential qualities

There are certain attributes that you should be able to discuss from your work experience. These can be divided into those qualities which you have witnessed in others and those which you have demonstrated yourself. Opportunities to observe and demonstrate these qualities will vary by the type of placement, however, some important qualities that you should be able to discuss from your work experience include:

- **Teamwork.** This is essential because doctors do not work unaccompanied; indeed, the management of patients is becoming increasingly interdisciplinary. Doctors commonly

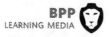

work alongside fellow doctors, nurses, physiotherapists, occupational therapists and social workers.

- **Leadership**. This is vital to the role of a doctor as you will often be expected to take the lead role in clinical situations and will be tasked with making important decisions regarding patients' management.
- **Empathy**. This is imperative because you will be dealing with people and their feelings. Studies show that patients are more likely to attend clinics and adhere to medication regimes if their doctor is able to show high levels of empathy.
- **Understanding the role of a doctor**. It is crucial that you are able to confidently discuss the role of a doctor in a clinical environment, in general and specific terms. This is fundamental in showing you have a realistic expectation of what a career in Medicine entails.
- **Professionalism**. Demonstrating high levels of professional behaviour is critical to becoming a doctor due to the high levels of responsibility and the public's high regard for the medical profession.

Remember that this is not an exhaustive list, but rather an indication of the types of areas you should aim to cover from your work experience. If you feel that you are not demonstrating these attributes through your existing placements, you may need to consider supplementing these with additional work experience.

What is the most valuable type of work experience?

Having discussed why work experience is important, the different types of work experience you may consider will now be discussed. You will not be expected to undertake work experience in all of the areas described below, however, you should attempt to gain sufficient experience to develop all of the above qualities.

You are applying to study a degree that will involve being in close contact with the public. It is therefore advisable to undertake experience in a healthcare environment that will expose you to healthcare professionals dealing with patients who are unwell. With many of the suggested forms of work experience you may need to have a CRB check. This can take some time to obtain, so plan well in advance to enable you to undertake the work experience prior to applying to medical school. Work experience can take many forms and the following are descriptions of the most common types.

Shadowing

A popular form of work experience is observing a doctor in their daily activities, which is known as shadowing. This is a very useful way of gaining firsthand experience of a doctor's specific duties in caring for patients. In addition to this, you are also likely to receive the opportunity to observe other tasks performed by doctors in a typical day, such as teaching junior colleagues and medical students, attending meetings and completing administrative tasks. Shadowing, by its very nature, requires professionalism and maturity.

You will need to be proactive and organised to arrange this type of work experience. A good starting point is to enquire at your local health centre whether any General Practitioners in your area would be willing to let you shadow them. You might also find it useful to look in the Directory Enquiries for local health centres, or visit local NHS trusts websites.

Once you have identified a doctor who would be happy to be contacted, you should write to them stating that you are interested in becoming a doctor and would like to learn more about the role. The letter should explain why you want become a doctor and your availability. It is also advisable to enclose your current CV in order to demonstrate your academic record and previous work experience. You may also want to consider including a recommendation from a lecturer or previous employer to help you to secure a placement. Do not be disheartened if your first attempts to obtain work experience are not successful, the hard work will be worthwhile when you secure a placement.

It can be difficult to ascertain how long you should spend shadowing a doctor, but in order to gain a full appreciation of the varied role, you should aim for a minimum of one week for each placement you organise. There are many different areas within Medicine to choose from, so choosing whether to undertake work experience in Geriatrics, Cardiology or Urology should be dependent on your personal preferences (and of course which doctors allow you to shadow them). Remember that your focus should not be to learn

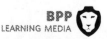

Medicine and Surgery in any great detail, but rather to experience the daily activities of a doctor and become familiar with some of the issues they face, with the aim that you should be able to discuss these with confidence in your personal statement or interview.

Hospital volunteering

Many NHS trusts will have vacancies for potential volunteers to spend time on the wards with patients. As a volunteer, activities you are likely to be involved in include delivering refreshments and talking to patients. While you will not be shadowing a doctor, you will gain valuable experience of hospital life. In particular, you will have an ideal opportunity to speak to patients and other healthcare professionals, such as nurses and healthcare assistants.

To find out more, you can locate your local NHS trust over the internet and apply for a volunteer position either through their website, or via telephone. You will be required to fill in an application form and may have to attend an interview, so be prepared to give the reasons why you want to volunteer. If you are interested in a particular area of Medicine you can state this on your application form and they may be able to arrange for you to be placed on a ward of that particular specialty. A CRB check will be undertaken which may take several weeks to be processed. Trusts will often expect a commitment of at least six months from volunteers, with a minimum of three hours per week.

Hospice volunteering

Hospices provide care for patients with serious, long term, and often terminal conditions. Patients often have a complex range of needs requiring both physical and psychological support. Generally, hospices are either nursing homes or hospitals, but they can also provide care within a patients' home. Hospices may be publicly or privately funded (or a combination of both) and are often in need of volunteers. While this sort of environment can be mentally and physically demanding, it provides an excellent insight into whether you are suited to a career in Medicine and whether you can cope with its demands. A good starting point for finding out how you may be able to get involved is the charity Help the Hospices.

Paid employment

If it is possible and you have enough time, you can undertake paid employment within the healthcare field. While there will always be competition for these roles, there are various jobs available that require limited, or no previous experience. Jobs that you may want to consider include healthcare assistant, phlebotomist, hospital porter and support worker. These jobs often require a commitment of at least 16 hours per week, so they may only be applicable if you are taking a gap year prior to your application. However, one advantage of this type of job is that work is often available through an agency which provides greater flexibility, allowing you more time to dedicate towards your application, or other commitments.

Job application forms can be surprisingly difficult to complete correctly and impress potential employees, so it may be worthwhile having a local careers adviser check that your application is both accurately completed and noteworthy. There are often more applications than jobs available so it is best to apply early. To find out the types of jobs available through the NHS jobs website.

Befriending services

Working for an organisation like ChildLine, Samaritans or SANE in providing support to vulnerable people can help to significantly improve communication and empathetic skills. It is also a good way to demonstrate your appreciation of medical ethics, such as patient confidentiality. Working for one of these organisations requires a longer term commitment than other placements, as training is required to attain the appropriate level of knowledge to undertake the role. For example, volunteering with Samaritans typically requires a commitment of six months. If you are interested in this form of work, useful contact details are provided at the end of the chapter.

Working with people with disabilities

You may have an interest in working with adults or children with learning or physical difficulties. This can either be on a voluntary basis, or as paid work. This type of job can present you with opportunities to enhance your interpersonal skills as some individuals may not be able to respond using typical forms of communication, and so other forms are required.

This type of job can be very challenging and may require providing personal care, such as assistance in mobility, hygiene and feeding. Your duties will vary depending on the age group and type of disability of the people you are looking after. A typical day may involve taking patients on outings to the cinema or playing simple sports games. Types of organisations that offer these services depend on your locality and to find these services it is advisable to contact your local council office. Similarly, a search on the internet should yield many local opportunities in this field.

Working in a nursing home

Spending time in a nursing home offers an excellent opportunity to see the complexities of providing care to older individuals and to learn that there is more to a patient than their illnesses. You will witness firsthand the challenges of treating individuals with multiple medical problems, such as managing a complex medical regime involving multiple drugs. You will also see the variety of physical and mental conditions which affect the elderly. This is also a fantastic way of developing your interpersonal and empathetic skills, as to gain the most from this experience you will need to communicate with many patients. When trying to organise a placement at a nursing home, the best method is to contact local nursing homes and enquire whether there are any opportunities to volunteer.

Working with younger children

Working with younger children can be an enjoyable experience and an excellent way to enhance your communication skills. This can prove to be very challenging, but if you are interested in pursuing a medical career with close contact with young children, such as Paediatrics or General Practice, this will be a particularly useful experience. Your local play group scheme can provide more information on how to pursue work experience in this field.

Reflecting on your experiences

To gain the most from volunteering and work experience you should try to record your daily experiences. You should record the tasks that you have undertaken, what you have learnt, and any areas that you may want to read more about to gain a clearer understanding of the subject. This will prove to be extremely useful when writing your personal statement and when preparing for your medical school interviews. It is valuable to write down not only the events, but how you felt and what you learnt from certain experiences. This is particularly valuable for situations that made an impression on you, as the details of such events can often be forgotten or distorted over time. When recording your experiences remember to maintain confidentiality and never to record a patient's identity.

Being able to recall experiences gained from work experience forms a major part of the assessment criteria and being able to discuss these will enhance your application. Reflective learning is an important part of undergraduate and postgraduate medical training and by showing that you have already developed this ability demonstrates to the admissions officer that you recognise the importance of this skill. Keeping a reflective diary is a highly useful tool for recording events during your work experience. Below is an excerpt from an example of a diary:

Event	Learning point
Day One – Spoke to Mrs X about her operation. While she was worried about her operation she was more concerned about who was looking after her pets at home.	Being a doctor is more than dealing with a patient's disease.
Day Two – Spent time shadowing one of the junior doctors. Today involved lots of cannulas, paper work, chasing X-rays and gathering notes.	Find out the career path for newly qualified doctors after they finish medical school.
Day Three – The consultant had to break bad news to a patient's family.	Being a good doctor involves more than being able to pass exams!

Extra-curricular activities

As well as work experience, extra-curricular activities form an important role in the application process for medical school and are an excellent way to demonstrate some of your personal characteristics, such as teamwork and professionalism. Just as importantly they show that you have interests outside of Medicine.

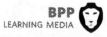

This is particularly essential as Medicine is a demanding career choice and extra-curricular activities display your ability to balance your time appropriately between your academic work and your other interests. Not everyone will be able to play sport at a national level or be the next Picasso; however the key thing is to participate in those activities that interest you and to gain something useful out of the experience. Below are some of the major skills that you should try to demonstrate through your extra-curricular activities:

- Teamwork
- Leadership
- Communication
- Responsibility
- Time management
- Organisation
- Negotiation
- Teaching

Fundraising for charitable organisations

This can be particularly fun, creative and worthwhile. There are many charities that require volunteers to fundraise (see the sections on volunteering for hospices and befriending services for more information). Ways in which you could help to fundraise include street campaigns, telephone campaigns or even holding a local street party, the list is endless.

One of the most common ways of fundraising is to participate in a walkathons or sponsored run. They range from 3k runs to marathons and are a great way of keeping fit! In addition, as one off events they do not require a major commitment. Although these experiences do not directly lead to patient contact, they are an excellent way to learn more about the work of medical charities and the conditions that they support.

Playing a sport or learning a new hobby

Joining a sports team offers exciting opportunities to meet new people and to keep healthy at the same time. This can be very useful way to display your ability to work in a team, as well as to demonstrate your work and well-roundedness. There are a whole range of sports that are available – try attending a local gym or sports centre, or having a look in the local advertisements in a newspaper or your local council office for more opportunities. Another avenue is to explore the opportunities available at various evening classes in your local area, as these activities may enable you to learn new skills, for example, art classes. Learning a new hobby can further demonstrate that you are a well-rounded person.

As is the case with gaining work experience, extra-curricular activities should be enjoyable. You should never feel that you must join a society or a team to have something to write on a medical school application, and if this is the case it will be transparent to many admissions tutors at an interview. Also, remember that there is no need to join every society or team available, as this will be counterproductive by occupying much of your time. Ultimately, joining a society should not be so demanding so as to negatively affect your academic grades. Being able to organise your time is a vital skill that admissions panels are looking for because of the time pressures exerted on both medical students and doctors.

Summary

- Well planned and carefully considered work experience can provide a significant advantage in your application.
- Work experience forms an essential part of the application process to medical school – choose the most appropriate form of work experience in order to gain the most from it.
- Although there are various types of work experience that you may wish to undertake, the skills you should be able to demonstrate through it are universal to all. These include (among others):
  - understanding the importance of empathy
  - the role of a doctor
  - leadership
  - professionalism.
- Different universities will recommend varied lengths of time to gain these skills; however consider whether you can confidently state that you have gained the most out of this experience.

- In addition to work experience, extra-curricular activities can display many other qualities that are required of a doctor and will thus form an integral part of the application process.

 Useful resources

www.jobs.nhs.uk
www.nspcc.org.uk
www.samaritans.org
www.childline.org.uk
www.sane.org.uk
www.helpthehospices.org.uk

Chapter 7
Admissions tests

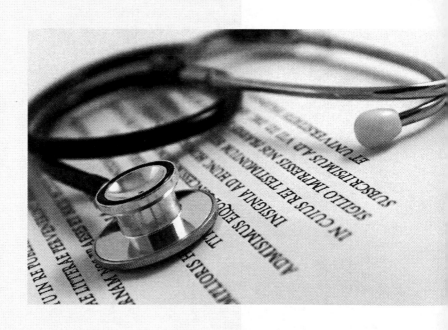

Admissions tests

Introduction

The past decade has seen growing concern from UK medical schools that A level exams are failing to adequately distinguish between candidates applying to study Medicine. As a result, most universities now employ admissions tests as a component of their selection process for entry into medical school. The extent to which these tests are utilised in the selection process differs between universities; with some choosing to use a candidate's test score in conjunction with their UCAS application to shortlist applicants for interview and others choosing to set specific test scores that must be met in order to be eligible for an interview. Unfortunately, graduates are not exempt from this process.

The three admissions tests used by UK medical schools are the UK Clinical Aptitude Test (UKCAT), the Graduate Australian Medical School Admissions (GAMSAT) and the Biomedical Aptitude Test (BMAT), which are all designed to test a candidate's critical thinking and problem solving skills. However, each test approaches this process in a different way, with the GAMSAT and BMAT designed to assess knowledge of Science and Maths, whereas the UKCAT is designed to avoid assessing prior knowledge in any subject.

What follows is a description of each of the admissions tests including an overview of their content, important test dates, and tips on exam preparation to give you the best chance of success.

The UKCAT

What is the UKCAT?

The UKCAT is the most widely used entrance exam for entry into medical schools in the UK. It is designed to assess a number of cognitive skills and competencies, such as decision-making and problem-solving, without assessing applicants' prior knowledge. The exam is completed at a test centre where applicants complete the exam on a designated computer. Prior to the exam, applicants must register on the UKCAT website where they are able to specify the test centre and time slot for their examination. The test is

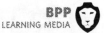

accessible around the world through various Pearson testing centres. For specific guidance regarding registering and sitting the test, it is recommended that applicants visit the UKCAT website.

Content of the UKCAT

The UKCAT does not test strict scientific or academic knowledge that may be found on an A level syllabus. Instead, it is designed to measure general mental abilities and behavioural attributes that are considered valuable in the medical or dental profession. Applicants are provided with a white board and pen and a simple on-screen calculator is available for performing calculations. The UKCAT is divided into four subtests:

1. **Verbal reasoning** – Assesses the candidate's ability to critically evaluate passages of written information covering a broad range of topics, including scientific and non-scientific themes. This subtest specifically tests an applicant's ability to interpret information from the text, rather than prior knowledge they may have on the topic.
2. **Quantitative reasoning** – Assesses the candidate's ability to analyse and manipulate complex numerical data, which has been adjusted to be appropriate to real life scenarios. This subtest requires knowledge of basic mathematical topics, including multiplication, division, percentages, and fractions.
3. **Abstract reasoning** – Assesses the candidate's ability to solve abstract problems. Specifically, it tests the ability to infer relationships between groups of shapes and to apply these rules to test shapes using divergent and convergent thinking.
4. **Decision analysis** – Assesses the candidate's quality of decision-making in terms of accuracy, adequacy, and time taken to arrive at a decision. This is measured by providing codes that must be translated and interpreted.

Non-cognitive analysis was a fifth section that was previously used to identify attributes and characteristics that contribute towards success in either Medicine or Dentistry, such as robustness, empathy, and integrity. However, this section was removed for the 2011 session.

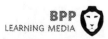

The test is presented in a multiple-choice format, whereby you must attempt to select the correct answer from a selection of distracters. Applicants have a set time in which to complete each subtest and any time remaining is not added to the subsequent subtest. The Verbal reasoning subtests is assigned 22 minutes, the Quantitative reasoning is assigned 23 minutes, the Abstract reasoning subtest is assigned 16 minutes, and the Decision analysis subtest is assigned 32 minutes.

Each subtest is scored individually on a scale of 300 to 900 and provided to the medical schools you apply to. Most applicants score between 500 and 700, with the average being 600. There is no pass rate for the UKCAT, instead the medical schools will review your result as part of your whole application, including your personal statement and academic grades. Each medical school has its own approach in how it uses the UKCAT result during the selection process.

Who requires the UKCAT and how to register

The UKCAT is used by 7 of the 16 GEM courses. These are:

- Barts and The London
- Imperial College London
- King's College London
- Leicester
- Newcastle
- Oxford
- Warwick

There is no single date for sitting the annual UKCAT exam and you are encouraged to check the key date on the UKCAT website. You should also try to book a test slot as soon as possible to improve your chances of attending a convenient test centre and time. There is a cost associated with taking the exam; however, this is reduced if the exam is taken early in the testing period. In 2011:

- If you sat the test between 5 July and 31 August the test fee was £65 (£100 if taken outside of the European Union)
- If you sat the test between 1 September and 7 October the test fee was £80 (£100 if taken outside of the European Union)

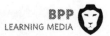

If you do not sit the exam by the last testing date of the year you will be ineligible to apply to medical schools which use the UKCAT. It is also important to note that if your application to your chosen medical school is unsuccessful and you decide to reapply the following year, you will be required to sit the UKCAT again.

There is also a UKCAT Special Educational Needs (SEN) version of the exam, which is identical except that additional time is allowed for completion of the test. It is designed for individuals with special circumstances, such as a disability or illness.

Preparing for the UKCAT

Candidates are encouraged to carefully read through the UKCAT website to gain a clear understanding of the test process, and to become familiar with the test interface used in the test centres.

The UKCAT website states that you cannot prepare for the UKCAT, however this is not strictly true – while the content of the test cannot be anticipated, familiarity with the layout of each of the subtests will facilitate better time management and speed. Therefore practice questions are a must. The first place for practice should be the UKCAT website, which provides a practice test in different formats: regular timing, not timed, short, and SEN. More comprehensive resources are available that allow extensive practice at the types of questions you will be expected to answer:

- **Books** – A large range of books is available which will guide you through the four subtests of the exam. This information will be selective and focus your learning to provide the best chance of equipping you with the skills to score highly
- **Online** – A number of websites provide online courses delivering very similar information to that found in the books previously mentioned, however, the information may be presented in a way that closely matches the format you will be presented with at the testing centre
- **Study courses** – Courses are available for applicants to attend in person. These courses typically discuss techniques for performing well and also offer mock examinations under test conditions. An added benefit is the access to a teacher who may be able to offer advice on areas you are having particular difficulty with.

 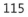

Tips for success in the UKCAT

Start your preparation early. Read through the UKCAT website carefully as soon as possible to avoid missing deadlines or falling behind schedule with your preparation.

Complete as many practice questions as you can prior to sitting the test. Completing many practice questions will make you more familiar with the test, faster at completing questions, and less nervous in the exam.

Register online and book a slot early. Delaying booking a slot may result in the inconvenience of having to travel further to a test centre, or potentially missing your slot completely. A further benefit is that you will save money by booking sooner rather than later.

Do not spend too much time on any one question. You will have a limited amount of time per section, so do not waste time on questions you are unsure of. The test allows you to 'flag' questions that you plan to return to.

Work to the clock. Pace judgement is crucial. Through practice you will develop the ability to accurately gauge how long to spend on each question before moving on.

As you will only be awarded marks for correct answers and there is no negative marking, **always answer every question**.

The GAMSAT

What is the GAMSAT?

The GAMSAT examination was developed by the Australian Council for Educational Research (ACER), however, it is now employed by a number of UK medical schools offering graduate entry programmes.

The GAMSAT is similar to the UKCAT in that it is designed to assess general cognitive skills, such as problem-solving and critical thinking; however, it differs in several important aspects. Unlike the UKCAT, the test also assesses knowledge of scientific

BPP
LEARNING MEDIA

concepts, and therefore revision is advisable to achieve your best performance. Also, unlike the UKCAT, the GAMSAT is a paper, rather than computer based exam, and questions consist of both multiple choice and essay questions.

All of the medical schools that employ the GAMSAT consider graduates with either Science, or non-Science degrees. Therefore, if you are a non-Science graduate applying to Graduate Entry Medicine, there is a good chance that you will be required to sit the GAMSAT. The questions in the Science section of the test are set at A level and early degree level. If your first degree was non-scientific, you will need to invest in some time to revise for the Science section, however, do not be too disheartened as every year many applicants with a previous degree in the Humanities or Arts are successful with their applications.

Content of the GAMSAT

Questions are based on a variety of sources. Typically, you will be asked to read a passage of writing and then be asked to answer questions about it. You will also be required to apply your knowledge of Biology, Chemistry, and Physics when interpreting information presented in numerical and graphical form.

The GAMSAT is divided into three sections:

1. **Reasoning in the Humanities and Social Sciences** – Focuses on assessing your problem-solving capabilities in a wide range of subjects. You will be presented with different kinds of information, usually in text form, but also in the form of an image or table. This information will deal with a range of public and academic issues, with an emphasis on socio-cultural and personal topics. The information provided will be used as subject matter for a series of questions. Each question will be presented in a multiple-choice format, with four alternative answers to choose from. This section contains 75 questions and you will be given 10 minutes' reading time, followed by 100 minutes to complete the questions.

2. **Written communication** – This section will test your essay writing skills. It is used to investigate your imaginative capabilities, as well as how able you are to express your ideas in writing. You will be provided with a number of

 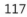

general ideas (usually quotes), relating to an overall theme. There will be two themes and you must complete two 30-minute essays, one on each theme. This section is assessed on two criteria: first, the thought and content of your work (that is, the quality of what you have written) and second, the organisation and expression of your work (that is, the fluency of the language and the accuracy of the grammar).

3.   **Reasoning in Biological and Physical Sciences** – This section examines knowledge of basic scientific concepts in addition to problem-solving within a scientific context. Content material is provided using various formats. Tasks you may be asked to perform include generating hypotheses, analysing data, discovering relationships and estimating measurements. Questions in this section cover Chemistry, Biology (which account for 40% of the total questions each) and Physics (which accounts for the remaining 20%). In order to answer these questions you should be comfortable with A level Physics and first year degree level Chemistry and Biology. This section contains 110 multiple-choice questions. You will be given 10 minutes' reading time and 170 minutes to answer the questions. This section contributes half of the total marks in the exam.

The GAMSAT score

You will receive a score for each section, plus an overall score based on the three sections. Sections I and II contribute 25% each, and section III contributes 50% towards the overall mark. The score is given on a scale of 1 to 100, however it is worthwhile to note that it is not a percentage score. Medical schools vary in how they use your GAMSAT score in the admissions process. Some will set a threshold that must be attained in order to be considered for interview, while others will use your score in conjunction with other information, such as your personal statement.

Unlike the UKCAT score, which is only valid for one year, the GAMSAT score is valid for two years. Therefore, if you take the exam in any one academic year and are unsuccessful in gaining a place, your score will still be valid the following year.

Who requires the GAMSAT and how to register

Currently there are four graduate entry courses in the UK that require applicants to take the GAMSAT. These are:

- Keele
- Nottingham
- St George's
- Swansea

Unlike the UKCAT, which can be taken any time during the testing period, all applicants sitting the GAMSAT UK sit the test on the same day. You are advised to go to www.gamsat.org.uk to check the key dates. In 2011, registration cost £195 with an additional fee of £50 applying to those who registered late. GAMSAT test centres are located in the following cities:

- Bristol
- London
- Nottingham
- Sheffield
- Swansea
- Melbourne, Australia

There are a limited number of places for candidates at each venue and places are allocated on a first come basis, therefore it is important to register early. If you suffer from any disability that may interfere with your ability to take the test, you must follow the instructions provided on the GAMSAT website on applying for Special Testing Consideration. It is strongly recommended that candidates familiarise themselves with this website and read through it carefully, as it provides the most up to date information on current deadlines.

Preparing for the GAMSAT

Most candidates find the third section of the exam the most intimidating, and therefore focus their efforts on revising Science and Maths. This is understandable given its large contribution toward the overall score; however it is not advisable to attempt to revise the entire A level syllabuses of Biology, Chemistry, Physics, and Maths. Instead it may be more beneficial to proceed directly to practice questions – an excellent starting point is the practice

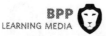

questions available to purchase on the GAMSAT website. After you have completed some practice questions you will have a far clearer idea of which topics you will need to focus your study on. Once you have identified any areas of weakness, you should seek out the modality of revision that suits you best, these include:

*   **Books** – A large range of books are available which will guide you through the key aspects of each of the core subjects. Arguably, the best source of practice questions are those provided by ACER, the developers and co-ordinators of the test. A book of sample and practice questions will cost £16, while a practice test book will cost £26. A level Science revision books are also a good way of equipping yourself with the knowledge to score highly in the third section of the exam.
*   **Online** – A number of websites provide online courses delivering very similar information to that found in the books, however, these sources claim to deliver the information in a more interactive manner, thereby helping you to retain the information.
*   **Study courses** – Some companies in the UK are now providing courses for applicants to attend in person. These will give you an idea of the necessary information over the course of a few days. These courses have the benefit of providing you with access to a well-informed teacher who may be able to explain concepts that are more difficult to grasp.

Tips for success in the GAMSAT

*   **Do not neglect your essay writing skills**. A little practice can be very useful in improving your writing, such as resolving basic grammar problems.
*   **Read through the GAMSAT website carefully** and know what is expected of you for each section of the exam.
*   Use practice questions to **identify any weak areas** and focus your study on these areas.
*   Set out a **study timetable** for each section so that you do not fall behind schedule. This can happen very easily, particularly if you are studying for two separate admissions tests.
*   **Do not waste time** on the internet trying to find the score that will get you shortlisted for interview. Knowing what score

you require will not help you to reach this target. Instead, work as hard as you can on getting the best score you can.

The BMAT

What is the BMAT?

The BMAT is owned and administered by Cambridge Assessment, who are also responsible for producing and marking the test. It is used by some UK universities in the selection process for candidates applying to Medicine, as well as Pharmacology, Veterinary Science, and Biomedical Sciences. Designed to make it easier for universities to differentiate between applicants with similar academic grades, the BMAT focuses on assessing problem-solving and critical thinking. This test assesses prior knowledge up to GCSE level Maths and Science. Therefore, only a minimal amount of revision is required. The BMAT is a written exam using multiple choice and essay format questions.

Content of the BMAT

The BMAT is a two-hour written exam, consisting of three sections. Calculators and dictionaries are not permitted in the exam. There are three parts to the BMAT:

1. **Aptitude and skills** – Contains three types of question, which assess problem-solving, understanding and argument, and data analysis and inference. It is one hour long and contains 35 questions, mostly multiple choice but also some short answer questions.
2. **Scientific knowledge and applications** – Designed to test core knowledge in Science and Maths up to GCSE level. Applicants have 30 minutes to complete 27 questions, which consist of predominantly multiple choice, but also some short answer questions.
3. **Writing task** – Assesses applicants' ability to develop ideas and communicate them clearly and effectively. Applicants are given 30 minutes to produce an essay style answer to one of four questions. Typically these questions will be based on a statement or short extract.

Who requires the BMAT?

If you are applying for a four-year Graduate Entry Medicine programme it is not a requirement that you take the examination for any of the courses. However, the University of Cambridge will consider BMAT scores within an application. The BMAT exam is of particular relevance to graduates applying to Undergraduate Medicine, where it is currently required by the following institutions:

- Imperial College London
- University of Cambridge
- University College London
- University of Oxford

Registration and important dates

Unlike the UKCAT and GAMSAT, you must register with a BMAT centre in order to sit the exam. Traditionally, your school or college would do this for you, however as a graduate you must contact your local centre directly, which can be located by visiting the Cambridge assessment website. There is a cost associated with taking the exam and a late registration fee may also be applied. In 2011:

- Registration with a UK/EU BMAT centre between 1 and 30 September cost £42.50 (£72.50 if taken outside of the EU).
- Registration with a UK/EU BMAT centre between 1 and 14 October incurred an additional £30 late entry fee.

All applicants take the exam on the same day annually. In 2011, the test date was 2 November and results were released on 23 November. As with the other admissions tests, places at test centres are limited and early registration is necessary to guarantee your place at a convenient location. BMAT results are only valid for one year and therefore you will have to re-sit the exam the following year if your application is unsuccessful. Furthermore, the test centre you register with may also add an administration fee.

Tips for success in the BMAT

- It is important that you **register early** so that you can attend a centre near you, which will allow you to arrive relaxed and on time.
- The BMAT is a difficult exam in which **preparation is paramount**. Most students find completing the questions within the allocated time the most challenging aspect. The best way to improve your exam technique is to practise under test conditions. Consider investing in a book or course.
- Focus your **preparation on weak areas**. Most candidates find the Scientific Knowledge and Application section the most demanding section. Therefore, practise your basic Mathematics skills to improve your accuracy and speed. You may be surprised at how little you have used these skills since your previous degree!
- Most universities consider your score as part of your whole application; so **do not neglect other aspects of your application** such as the personal statement.

 Summary

- Most Medical Schools use information from aptitude tests to arrive at a decision about your application for Graduate Entry Medicine, so it is likely that you will have to sit at least one of these exams.
- For the entrance exams you will be sitting, it is important to know:
  - key dates
  - subject matter
  - preparation techniques.
- Use the information above to help with your planning and get down to work as soon as possible.
- Preparation for these tests is vital, but remember you probably will not begin studying until you have a test date booked so do this as soon as possible.

 Useful resources

www.ukcat.ac.uk
www.gamsatuk.org
www.admissionstests.cambridgeassessment.org.uk/adt/bmat

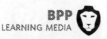

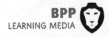

Chapter 8
The Medical School interview

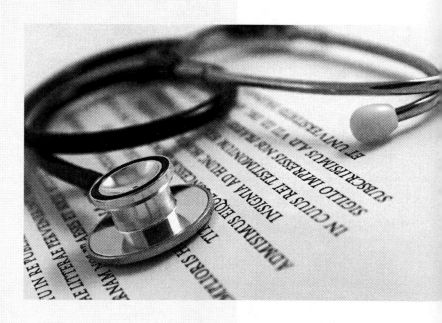

The Medical School interview

In order to gain a place at medical school you must be able to demonstrate more than merely academic excellence: you must possess something far less tangible – the qualities required to become a doctor. Due to the difficulty in determining many of these from the UCAS application alone, assessing these attributes is largely the business of the interview panel.

The aim of this chapter is to assist you in your preparation for interview by identifying the qualities the interview panels will be looking for, how they will be assessed at interview, and the format of the selection process. Guidance on improving your interview technique and practical aspects to be aware of for your interview are also covered in the chapter.

'Tomorrow's Doctors'

The GMC sets the standards and outcomes expected of a medical graduate in its document *Tomorrow's Doctors* (2009), and in turn medical schools are required to ensure that only the students that meet these standards are permitted to graduate. Therefore, it is within every medical school's interest to only select candidates who they believe have the potential to fulfil these outcomes. Indeed, many medical schools make explicit reference to this document in their selection criteria and statements. In addition to the scientific knowledge and practical skills required for clinical practice, the GMC highlights the importance of personal and professional values. These qualities are outlined in the document *The Doctor as a Professional* (within *Tomorrow's Doctors*, 2009) and those particularly relevant to the prospective student are summarised as follows:

- Be polite, honest and trustworthy and act with integrity.
- Show respect for others regardless of age, race, gender, sexual orientation, disability or religious beliefs.
- Show a commitment towards learning beyond the duration of the medical degree; medical knowledge is continuously changing and practice must be adapted accordingly.
- Demonstrate initiative, resilience and the ability to solve problems.

- Work safely as a doctor and recognise personal limitations and seek help where appropriate.
- Be able to prioritise tasks and effectively organise their time.
- Exhibit excellent communication skills when interacting with patients and other members of the medical team.
- Work effectively as both a leader and member of a team, particularly as medical care is increasingly co-ordinated through a multidisciplinary team.

The selection process

While all medical schools are essentially looking for the same qualities in a candidate, the means by which they do this varies considerably. Some medical schools continue to employ a traditional approach to interview, in which applicants are asked questions in front of an interview panel. In contrast, a number of other medical schools have adopted the more modern approach of using assessment centres. What follows is a summary of the interview formats at each of the 16 Graduate Entry Courses in the UK.

Barts and The London

Barts and the University of Warwick operate a joint admissions process; however they make independent decisions when offering places. Applicants are invited to attend a half-day selection centre where they are given a number of observed tasks to complete, including a written task, a group task, a personal interview and a feedback session. These tasks are designed to assess the degree to which applicants exhibit the qualities required to succeed in Medicine, and may take the form of written assessments, observation and evaluation of a patient consultation, teamwork exercises, as well as individual interviews. Each component is assessed according to pre-determined criteria.

University of Birmingham

At Birmingham, selection is based on a structured interview conducted by a panel of interviewers, which usually consists of the admissions tutor, a member of the teaching staff involved in the graduate course and a senior medical student. Interviews last 15 to 20 minutes. Questions are focused on the candidate's

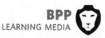

motivation towards a career in Medicine and whether they possess the essential merits required to succeed in such a career, using the personal statement as a starting point. There is an opportunity for the applicant to ask questions towards the end of the interview.

University of Bristol

At Bristol, selection is carried out via a 15- to 20-minute interview conducted by a panel of two interviewers. Interviewers are interested in establishing the applicants' motivations to study Medicine, what they understand about the structure of the course and medical careers, as well as their knowledge of recent medical developments. The Medical School highlights the personal qualities and skills needed to become a doctor in the section 'being a doctor' on its website.

University of Cambridge

In general, there are two interviews lasting 20 to 45 minutes each held on consecutive days. Therefore, an overnight stay at Cambridge is usually required. The form and length of the interview varies considerably at each college, therefore you are recommended to contact the college you are applying to for the exact format of the interview. Applicants are advised to research topics in the news related to Medicine, being particularly mindful of any recent medical developments.

Imperial College London

Interviews at Imperial are held by a panel consisting of a chairperson and two to four additional members, including a clinician and an academic, and often a lay person and a student. Interviews are typically 45 minutes in length and follow a semi structured format. The aim of the process is to evaluate the candidate's personal attributes, and in particular their motivation towards a career in Medicine. Emphasis is also placed on an understanding of mammalian cell biology. Therefore, if you have not been involved in active study recently, it may be worthwhile refreshing your memory of basic Biology.

Keele University

The interview at Keele Medical School lasts approximately 20 minutes and is carried out by a panel consisting of an academic, a clinician and a lay person, one of whom will have read your personal statement. Interviewers are interested in the applicant's abilities to communicate effectively and display some knowledge of current medical issues. Also, applicants should expect questions on their work experience and what they have learnt from it.

King's College London

King's employs the Multi Mini Interview (MMI) system. This involves candidates moving between eight stations, each lasting five minutes, where they are interviewed and marked independently by two interviewers. Questions focus on work experience and extra-curricular activities and emphasis is placed on demonstrating a commitment to Medicine. Interviews are conducted by clinicians and academics. Students not accepted onto the graduate entry course may be considered for the undergraduate course.

University of Leicester

From 2011, Leicester Medical School will be using the MMI system. Candidates will be assessed on their problem solving skills, written and verbal communication skills, and their motivation and commitment towards Medicine. Further details are still to be released. Candidates are encouraged to visit the 'admissions news' section of the medical school website for up to date information on the interview structure.

University of Liverpool

Candidates to Liverpool are invited to a 15-minute interview carried out by two interviewers drawn from a pool, which includes academic staff and clinicians, who may be either GPs or hospital doctors. Applicants should be aware of the Liverpool curriculum and the career pathway in Medicine, and have some appreciation of medical ethics. The candidate is scored independently by each interviewer, which contributes to an overall score.

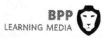

Newcastle University

At Newcastle, a structured interview is conducted by two interviewers drawn from a pool of academics, administrative staff, clinicians, healthcare professionals and lay selectors. Interviews last approximately 25 minutes. Interviewers are seeking candidates who demonstrate strong motivation and enthusiasm for pursuing a career in Medicine. Particular importance is placed on personal experience of interacting with people in a caring environment, and the ability to reflect on these and other experiences.

The University of Nottingham

Nottingham Medical School uses the MMI system, with three interviewers selected from clinicians, academics and lay persons. Lay people are drawn from professionals who work in health related subjects, such as the Health Sciences, Education and Human Resources. There are eight stations each lasting six minutes, with one or two interviewers present. Interviewees will be questioned about their knowledge of what a medical career entails and their personal interest in Medicine. Again, the selectors will be looking for personal attributes necessary for successful entry into the profession.

University of Oxford

Candidates attend two interviews at their chosen colleges; one focused on their application, achievements and ambitions, the other focussed on their problem-solving skills. It is also common to attend an additional interview at a different college. Interviews are conducted by tutors from the college and clinicians and last approximately 20 to 30 minutes. Emphasis is placed on academic ability and applicants may be asked scientific based questions. Personal suitability towards Medicine is also considered, as evidenced by strong communication skills, a mature attitude and well-developed organisational skills.

University of Southampton

Southampton Medical School does not generally interview graduate applicants, unless additional information is required beyond what is given on the UCAS form. If this is the case, the interview will be conducted by two members of staff who will have access to your personal statement. Each interviewer assesses the non-academic abilities and marks these out of a score of five. They are particularly interested in articulate individuals who demonstrate initiative and self-motivation, along with an ability to draw on their own personal experiences when asked.

St George's, University of London

St George's Medical School uses the MMI system. Applicants complete activities and interviews at seven stations, each lasting five minutes. These may include role play with an actor, practical tasks and answering interview questions. A number of examples are available on the St George's website.

Swansea University

Applicants to Swansea are interviewed to determine whether they possess the qualities required to become a doctor. The interview panel typically consists of clinicians and academics who are involved in teaching the course. Interviews are typically 30 minutes in length and follow a semi-structured format.

University of Warwick

Applicants attend a joint selection day with students who have applied to Barts and The London where they are given a number of observed tasks to complete over half a day, which include written assessments, team work exercises, personal interviews, observation, evaluation of a patient consultation and a feedback session. Each component is assessed according to predetermined criteria.

Interview questions

It is impossible to anticipate every question that may be asked at interview, but there are some subjects that consistently arise during medical school interviews. The types of questions most frequently asked can be split into three broad categories:

- Questions about your personal qualities and characteristics.
- Questions that assess your knowledge of medical topics.
- Questions that assess your ability to tackle ethical scenarios.

Each of these areas is explored in the next section.

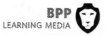

Through preparation for your medical school interview, your interview technique will improve and your confidence will increase, however, you should be wary of rote learning answers to common questions for two reasons. First, interviewers are seeking articulate individuals who are able to formulate responses under pressure; therefore appearing to have rehearsed your answers may create a negative impression. Second, having rehearsed answers to specific questions, it can be tempting to use those same answers to similar yet subtly different questions. Nonetheless, it can be helpful to think of some general responses for broad themes that can be tailored to answer a range of questions during the interview.

Finally, it is important to apply a systematic approach when answering questions. Remember that it is perfectly acceptable and even preferable to pause and collect your thoughts before answering. Try to be concise in your answer and address each part of the question in turn. If it is not clear what is being asked, seek clarification. Recognise that you will not be able to anticipate every question and some questions will be unexpected. Attempt to answer the question, but be honest if you do not know the answer as interviewers will soon realise if you are fabricating your answer.

Types of questions

Personal qualities and characteristics

As previously discussed, the interview panel will largely be concerned with identifying whether you have the necessary qualities and motivation to become a doctor. When answering questions designed to assess these characteristics, it is not enough to simply describe the qualities you possess; you must qualify them with examples. It is therefore worthwhile to consider your strengths and identify situations when you have demonstrated them, before the interview. It is also important to be aware of your weaknesses and how you have overcome them. This is particularly relevant in Medicine where a vital element of safe clinical practice is to recognise your own limitations. When contemplating your strengths and weakness, you may find it useful to write these down, or create a mind map to help structure your ideas before the interview.

You are also likely to be asked one or more questions regarding your personal statement; therefore it is a good idea to refresh your

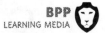

memory of what you wrote and consider any questions which could arise from it. An effective approach to preparing for questions on your personal statement is to enlist a friend or family member to ask you questions on what you have written.

'Why do you want to become a doctor?'

This is a favourite question of medical school interviewers and for good reason. Your answer can provide a great deal of information about your understanding of and suitability towards a career in Medicine. In your response you may wish to include any personal experiences that confirmed your decision to pursue a career in Medicine, such as work experience.

Furthermore, consider what Medicine offers you that alternative careers do not. It is fine as part of your answer to express your desire to help people, but as there are many jobs that provide this opportunity, you must be able to elaborate on this. For example, you might say that while all healthcare professionals are involved in the care of their patients, only doctors are able to use their knowledge and clinical experience to form a diagnosis; or that you are seeking a challenging career in a profession which offers many areas in which to specialise. Naturally, it would be unwise to offer financial or self-serving motivations as a reason.

'What qualities should a doctor have?'

This question closely relates to the qualities outlined in *Tomorrow's Doctors* (2009) such as a genuine interest in people, an open and enquiring mind, imagination, determination and an ability to work under pressure. Consider why these attributes are advantageous in a doctor, and if there are some that you believe are particularly important. You may even be able to reflect on a situation in which a doctor displayed one or more of these qualities during a work placement, or in your own personal experience.

'How do you cope with stress?'

Variations of this question commonly appear in interviews, as undertaking medical training and working as a doctor can be extremely demanding and stressful. It is probably not advisable to say that stress does not affect you, as stress is an almost universal experience, and furthermore, stress exists on a spectrum and an

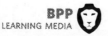

optimum amount actually improves performance. Think of times when you have been faced with challenging events and examine how you dealt with them. Identify what you found particularly difficult about the situation and what you would do differently if it were to occur again. Effective coping strategies you may have employed include pausing to review the situation, prioritising work, setting yourself deadlines and using relaxation techniques.

'What did you learn from your work experience?'

Medical schools expect prospective students to have performed some form of work experience. It is important to recognise that what you have gained from the experience is equally as important as the experience itself. If you are still undertaking voluntary work, it is helpful to record your thoughts and learning points in a diary. Alternatively, recall and reflect upon the defining moments of your work experience. For example, you may be able to identify an event which highlighted the importance of certain characteristics of a doctor, or perhaps you were involved in an emotionally difficult situation. Consider how you coped with this at the time and how you would approach it if faced with the same situation again. There may have been an aspect of the work that confirmed your interest in pursuing Medicine, such as helping a patient or witnessing an interesting case. The interviewers will be interested in whether you can reflect and learn from your experiences, as this plays an increasingly important role in Medicine.

Fact-based questions

All medical schools will assume that you have thoroughly researched the structure of their course and how it is taught, therefore you should expect to be asked questions about this. As a starting point, an overview of each course is given in Chapter 4. Other areas you will be expected to be familiar with include career progression as a doctor, the structure of the NHS and current affairs affecting the health service.

The NHS has an excellent medical careers website, which also provides plenty of advice for prospective students. The BBC news website also offers up to date and concise news on medical topics. Topics of particular interest include health resource allocation, the portrayal of Medicine in the media and the role of the National

Institute for Health and Clinical Excellence (NICE) in clinical practice. Also consider current health challenges, such as the impact of an aging population, high levels of obesity and hospital acquired infections, such as MRSA and *Clostridium difficile*. A summary of the structure of the NHS is provided by the NHS choices website, along with links to other useful information, including the role of NICE.

Finally, you may be interested in reading articles in medical literature: the *British Medical Journal*, the *New England Journal of Medicine* and *The Lancet* are some of the most well known and respected journals, and often publish articles that have significant impact on healthcare in the UK and abroad. Furthermore, some of their articles are open access and therefore do not require subscription to the journal. Most medical school interviewers will not ask you direct questions about your knowledge in the Sciences, however, there are some exceptions such as the University of Oxford and Imperial College London.

Ethics-based questions

Discussion based questions on ethical issues are popular with medical school interviewers as they allow them to observe your reasoning and communication skills. As is often the case in Medicine, there are often no right or wrong answers. When answering such questions try to provide a balanced argument and present the reasoning behind your viewpoint.

Interviewers may ask questions about medical ethics, such as confidentiality, either directly or (more likely) indirectly though an ethical scenario. It is not within the scope of this book to explore medical ethics in detail, nor will you be expected to have a full appreciation of it at this stage in your career. However, a basic understanding of the four principles used in medical ethics will provide a structure for your answer and a sound basis for your argument. The ethical principles are:

Autonomy

This is the principle of allowing individuals to arrive at a decision freely and independently. In the context of Medicine this requires doctors to provide the necessary information to help patients reach

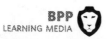

informed decisions and to respect the decisions made by patients, even if they do not agree with them. You could use the principle of autonomy to justify offering women the choice to terminate a pregnancy. Of course, in such a contentious debate it is always important to be aware of conflicting ethical arguments. In this case, that the foetus could be argued to be a person with rights of its own.

Beneficence

This is the principle of performing good acts and in the context of Medicine relates to doctors acting in the best interests of the patient at all times. Therefore, any procedure or treatment carried out on a patient should firstly be of direct benefit to the patient. However, difficulties lie in interpreting what is best for the patient. A patient may not agree with the doctor's opinion of what is best for them. Paternalism is where a doctor ignores the belief of a patient and acts in a way that he believes will most benefit the patient. This is a somewhat old fashioned approach to Medicine because greater emphasis is now placed on forming an alliance with the patient. In this way, beneficence should be balanced with autonomy.

Non-maleficence

This is the principle of not doing wrong and in the context of Medicine relates to doctors avoiding harm to their patients. It is therefore closely related to the principle of beneficence. When you consider medical treatments, they all confer a degree of potential harm, in terms of side effects and risks. Therefore, it is common that a compromise is sought to ensure the benefits of the treatment outweigh the risks involved. Difficulties arise when the doctor and patient have different ideas about what the benefit may be and how acceptable the risks, or side effects, are. Not taking into account a patient's view could result in the doctor causing greater harm than they realise, despite the doctor believing they are behaving in the patient's best interest.

Justice

This principle relates to the idea of universal fairness and in the context of Medicine is of particular significance when considering how medical resources should be allocated. The principle of justice comes into play in the arguments surrounding the so called 'postcode lottery', which refers to discrepancies in access to healthcare for patients under the care of different Primary Care Trusts. You may argue that this defies the principle of justice because people unfairly receive different treatment based purely on where they live. Alternatively, it may be argued that resources are allocated differently in each trust according to the needs of that population and this may differ from neighbouring trusts.

Practical issues

It may seem like common sense but it is important to not only prepare for the types of questions you may be asked, but also the practical aspects of your interview. This will reduce the possibility of any problems occurring during the interview and also help to reduce the amount of stress you experience on the day. Make your travel arrangements early and ensure you have ample time for travelling. It is much better to arrive early and wait, than to rush and risk being late. If you have not been sent a map with the location of the medical school, check the respective university's website as many feature a map. If you require any information regarding the interview that has not been provided, this should be sought in advance by contacting the medical school via email, telephone or in person.

It is also important to prepare the clothes you plan to wear to the interview in advance – a suit or smart trousers, with a shirt and tie is advisable for men, while women should wear a conservatively cut shirt with trousers or a skirt, which should be at least knee length. You should ensure that you appear clean and presentable, and furthermore that your clothes are comfortable, as any discomfort can be reflected in your body language and speech.

Body language

It is important to be aware of your body language, as interviewers begin to form their impression of you from the moment you enter the room. Therefore, you should aim to project a professional and confident demeanour from the outset. Some useful tips to remember are to smile and acknowledge the panel at the start of the interview. Adopt a comfortable position, without appearing to slouch or look too casual, and during the interview place hands

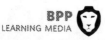

in your lap on the table to avoid crossing your arms, as this gives a defensive impression. While talking, make eye contact with the interviewers and address your answers to the whole panel. At the end of the interview, smile and thank the panel for their time. The key thing is to be yourself; it is you that the interview panel are interested in and not a persona that you think they will appreciate more. While you may feel under pressure it is important to try to relax during the interview as this will allow you to formulate ideas more easily and help you to express yourself naturally. If you are prone to nerves, a practical way to relax is to reframe the situation to one which evokes less anxiety. One way to achieve this is to try to perceive the interview as a conversation between you and the panel to decide, not only whether you are suited to the medical school, but also whether the medical school is suited to you. This should enable you to be less nervous at the interview, and to appear more confident and professional.

 ## Summary

- While academic achievements are important, the interview panel are also searching for candidates who possess the qualities required to become a doctor.
- These qualities are outlined in *Tomorrow's Doctors* and include among other attributes:
  - good communication skills
  - a commitment to lifelong learning
  - integrity of character
  - an interest in people.
- Medical Schools use different methods to evaluate candidates, from the traditional interview to the MMI system used in assessment centres.
- Regardless of the format, interviewers will ask questions to determine your motivation and suitability for a career in Medicine.
- The answers that you provide in interview should demonstrate that you understand the attributes needed to be a doctor and that you possess them.
- Knowledge and awareness of:
  - the course
  - career progression
  - current health issues

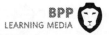

should help demonstrate that you have a genuine interest in Medicine and that you have made a measured decision to pursue it as a career.

- Your performance at interview will be significantly improved by appropriate preparation, coupled with a confident and professional body language.

 Useful resources

www.gmc-uk.org (*Tomorrow's Doctors*)
www.medicalcareers.nhs.uk/considering_medicine/introduction.aspx
www.bbc.co.uk/news/health/
www.nhs.uk/NHSEngland/thenhs/about/Pages/nhsstructure.asp
www.thelancet.com/
www.bmj.com/ (British Medical Journal)
www.nejm.org/ (New England Journal of Medicine)

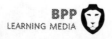

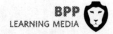

Chapter 9
Medical careers

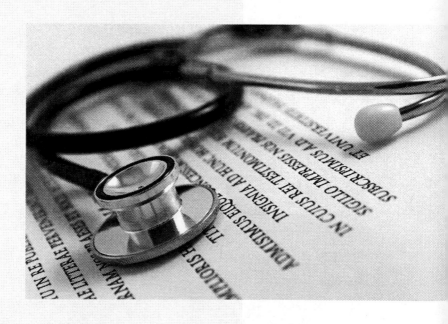

Medical careers

Completion of training to be able to work as a fully independent doctor takes a long time, and varies considerably by specialty. The career path of a doctor is guided by a programme called Modernising Medical Careers (MMC), which was launched in 2003 as an initiative to ensure that there was a national standard of career pathways for doctors. The aim of this was to enhance the quality of care for patients by reforming and improving postgraduate medical training and education.

As with other careers, many doctors may not end up in the same field that they aspired to when they first joined medical school. Try not to be alarmed by this; your ideal career is unique to you, shaped by your personal goals and desires. However, throughout life unexpected events can occur and priorities can alter, resulting in changes to your career aspirations. This chapter will outline the major stages in a medical career, as well as some of the most popular career pathways.

The Foundation Programme

After completing your journey through medical school, you will be provisionally licensed to the GMC as a newly qualified doctor, and will embark upon a two-year Foundation Programme. This Programme was introduced in 2005 as a bridge between medical school and specialty training, designed to equip newly qualified doctors with the generic professional and medical competencies required for effective and safe care of patients in the NHS.

Application to the Foundation Programme

Application to the Foundation Programme begins during your final year of studying Medicine, via a centralised application process which allocates new medical graduates to Foundation Programme placements across the UK. Details regarding the timeline of events for application are published on the UK Foundation Programme Office (UKFPO) website approximately six weeks before the application forms are released. The UKFPO publishes a handbook and timeline annually which is designed to help students with the application process. Based on their score and order of preference applicants are matched to a Foundation Programme to commence their training, provided they qualify from medical school and are provisionally registered with the GMC.

The Foundation Programme was over-subscribed for the first time for those applying to start in August 2011. In response to this, the UKFPO has developed a contingency plan for applicants who are not immediately allocated to a foundation school. This involves placing them on a reserve list and allocating them to a foundation school in batches as vacancies arise.

Selection to the Foundation Programme

Students applying to the Foundation Programme in 2013 and beyond will be selected using a new application system. The Situational Judgment Test will replace the current system of answering a series of short answer questions as a measure of meeting the professional attributes expected of a Foundation doctor. All applicants, including those applying to the Academic Foundation Programmes, will complete the test which is taken in exam conditions. Applicants must respond to a series of questions in one of two ways: either ranking five possible responses in the most appropriate order, or selecting the three most appropriate responses. The test consists of around 70 computer-marked questions and is completed in 2 hours and 20 minutes. A maximum of 50 points are available.

The Educational Performance Measure will replace academic quartiles as a measure of clinical and non-clinical skills, knowledge and performance up to the point of application. A maximum of 50 points are available. The score is comprised of three elements:

- Medical school performance (between 34 and 43 points available).
- Additional degrees (up to 5 points available).
- Academic achievements (up to 2 points available).

For further details on the changes to the application process, visit the Improving Selection to the Foundation Programme (ISFP) website.

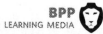

Objectives of Foundation training

As a new medical graduate undertaking foundation training there are several objectives you must meet during the course of your two years. These include the ability to:

- Confidently apply your clinical skills, particularly in the treatment of acutely-ill patients, in order to diagnose and care for seriously ill patients effectively.
- Display professional behaviour and attitudes in your clinical practice.
- Demonstrate competence in these areas through a thorough system of assessment.
- Explore a wide range of potential career pathways in different areas of Medicine.
- Meet the requirements for eligibility to apply for full registration with the GMC by the end of the first year of the Programme.

Foundation training is set within a structured and supervised two-year programme, based primarily in the workplace. The Foundation Programme Curriculum describes the outcomes that foundation doctors are required to demonstrate prior to completion of the first year (Foundation Year 1) and second year (Foundation Year 2) of the Foundation Programme.

Foundation Year 1

The first year of the Foundation Programme aims to build on the knowledge, competences and skills acquired during a medical degree. During each foundation year, doctors are required to complete rotations in various specialties. Foundation Year 1 will generally include at least three months of Medicine and three months of Surgery. Placements can vary in length, although three four-month placements are the most common.

Placements are designed to be long enough to allow foundation doctors to become integrated with the medical team, thus allowing senior doctors to be able to make reliable judgements on the abilities, performance and progress of the foundation doctor. In certain circumstances, it is possible for medical graduates to undertake their Foundation Year 1 training outside of the UK, however, you are advised to seek the advice of your medical school at an early stage if you are considering doing this.

In order to provide a record of their educational progress and achievements during the two years, foundation doctors are required to maintain an electronic portfolio. This is a vital document, as it is used for future job applications and interviews. Successful completion of Foundation Year 1 allows the doctor to apply for their full registration with the GMC and progress to Foundation Year 2.

Foundation Year 2

Foundation Year 2 expands on the first year of training, with the main focus on training in the assessment and management of acutely ill patients. Foundation Year 2 training also encompasses the generic professional skills that are applicable to all areas of Medicine, including communication, team work, time management and ICT skills. The most common framework for rotations during Foundation Year 2 is four three-month placements. Another major aim of these placements is to facilitate foundation doctors in making a well informed decision about the specialty training they wish to undertake upon completion of the Foundation Programme. It is possible to undertake your Foundation Year 2 year outside of the UK, however, for further information you should contact the foundation school or deanery in which you are due to complete your Foundation Year 1.

Satisfactory completion of the Foundation Programme requires foundation doctors to perform consistently well, and take on increasing levels of responsibility. This is to ensure that as a foundation doctor you are prepared for the next step in your medical career when you will commence your specialty training. On completion of Foundation Year 2, doctors are awarded the Foundation Achievement of Competence Document.

Specialty training

Following successful completion of the Foundation Programme the next stage of the career pathway is specialty training. This is the stage where doctors choose to pursue either a speciality in Medicine, Surgery or General Practice. It is often considered the

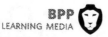

most crucial stage in a doctor's training, as progression through specialty training will allow doctors to gain competences that are required for them to act independently as a Consultant or General Practitioner. The decision to enter a particular specialty largely determines the career path for a doctor and therefore a great deal of thought and planning is required when making this decision.

Specialty training is provided through specialty training programmes and posts that are approved by the Postgraduate Medical Education and Training Board (PMETB). The length of training at this stage varies, and can take between three and eight years depending on the specialty chosen. This may also be extended if higher degrees or periods of research are undertaken. The PMETB approves the curriculum for speciality training programmes, which defines the standard of skills, knowledge and behaviours which must be demonstrated in order to progress through the training. Specialty training is organised into either a 'coupled' or 'uncoupled' training, which are detailed in the next section. Upon successful completion of a specialist training programme you will be awarded a Certificate of Completion of Training (CCT).

Uncoupled training

Uncoupled specialties are split into 'core' and 'higher' training. Core training is offered for two or three years, with core training years being referred to as CT1, CT2 and CT3. After core training, doctors must apply through open competition for higher specialty training posts, referred to as STS onwards, and can usually expect high levels of competition for these posts. If their application is successful, doctors continue in higher training for another four or five years, depending on the specialty until their CCT is awarded.

Coupled training

Coupled, or run-through training, allows the doctor automatic progression to the next level in their training, provided that competency requirements are satisfied. Run-through training is only offered by some specialties, see Table 9.1. In order to progress, doctors must pass assessments throughout the specialty training programme. Doctors must also achieve an Annual Review of Competence Progression in order to move through their training, until they are awarded their CCT. In addition, some run-through specialities offer other job opportunities and points of entry, such as one-year training posts called Fixed Term Specialty Training Appointments. These appointments allow doctors to gain more experience in an area before applying for a longer term position.

Uncoupled training in 2012	Run-through training in 2012
Anaesthesia	Obstetrics and Gynaecology
Core Medical Training	Ophthalmology
Core Surgical Training	Paediatrics and Child Health
Emergency Medicine	General Practice
Core Psychiatry Medicine	Public Health
	Neurosurgery
	Histopathology
	Chemical Pathology
	Medical Microbiology/Virology
	Clinical Radiology
	Academic Clinical Fellowship (ACF)

Table 9.1 Specialties offering uncoupled and run-through training

The flowchart in Figure 9.1 is an overview of the career structure for foundation and speciality training. It does not show all of the points of entry as these depend on the vacancies that become available at different stages of training.

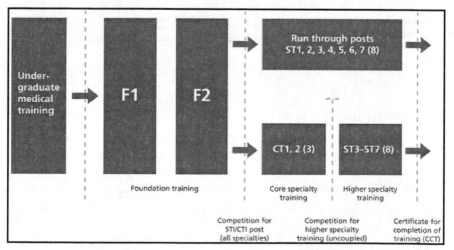

Figure 9.1 Overview of career structure for foundation and specialty training (diagram adapted from image by David Rice, KSS Deanery, 2008)

Application and competition for specialties

Specialty training application is completed via an online process. Application dates are released along with timelines to assist doctors with the application process. Doctors can make as many applications to different specialties as they wish, provided that they meet the competences and eligibility criteria for the post that they are applying for. There is huge variation in the number of training posts available in each specialty, as well as the popularity of the different specialties. When considering your specialty choice, you are recommended to consider the competition ratio for posts, which is based on the number of applicants for each post. Competition for different posts can be highly variable and tends to be influenced by factors such as geographical location and the changing trends in healthcare. For example, an increasing elderly population has resulted in the expansion of medical jobs in primary care, whilst the number of posts in certain surgical specialties has decreased.

As an applicant to specialist training you are advised to plan your applications carefully, and be prepared to be flexible in the event that you are unsuccessful in gaining a place on your first choice of specialty.

Membership exams and completion of specialist training

In order to progress to Consultant level, doctors must pass the membership and fellowship exams for the particular specialty that they intend to pursue. These exams are devised by a variety of Royal Colleges and are widely considered to be the most challenging exams you will face in your medical career. Membership exams are taken when entering specialist training and the fellowship exams are taken when a doctor nears completion of their specialist training. The exams consist of a number of parts and it is not uncommon for doctors to have to re-sit at least one part of the exam, reflecting the difficulty of the exams. An additional challenge arises from the need to combine a full time job with difficult academic revision.

Once a doctor completes their specialist training with a CCT award and passes the relevant fellowship exams, they are placed on the specialist register of the appropriate Royal College for their specialty. Doctors are then eligible to apply for Consultant or General Practitioner (GP) posts depending on the training pathway they have taken.

General Practice

General Practice is an extremely important part of Medicine throughout the world. General Practitioners (GPs) are usually the first point of contact for most medical services, either in a GP surgery or on a home visit. Around half of all medical students who qualify as doctors will eventually become GPs, with one of the major attractions being the range of clinical presentations seen. GPs simply cannot predict what they will be presented with next, which can be both stimulating and daunting. No other specialty available can offer such a wide variation in the medical conditions seen. A GP can provide a complete spectrum of care within a community, often dealing with problems that have physical, psychological, as well as social components. GPs require an extensive knowledge of medical conditions in order to be able to assess a problem, diagnose and determine an appropriate course of action. They decide when and how to intervene, not only through treatment, but also through education and prevention. For example, the role of the GP in disease prevention involves helping patients take responsibility for their own health and also the health of the patients' families.

Not only do GPs see a wide variety of patients, but they can also work in very different ways. GPs in England are grouped together in primary care trusts (PCTs), which consists of several GP surgeries and clinics, as well as other healthcare professionals, such as Pharmacists and Opticians. Many GPs are self-employed and hold contracts with the PCT, either independently or as part of a partnership. Almost all GPs work as part of a primary healthcare team, consisting of doctors, nurses, health visitors and administrative staff. This structure is under review at the time of writing due to the recent change in government. GPs are also increasingly working alongside other healthcare professionals such as nutritionists, speech therapists and physiotherapists. There are many opportunities for GPs in the UK, and also different types of practices which are outlined below.

- Group practices consist of a number of GPs in partnership. The administrative costs are shared between partners, and there is also the opportunity to share cases and problems within the group.
- Some GPs will chose to work without any medical partners, in single-handed practices. They often employ a nurse and

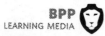

administrative staff. The main advantage of this is the ease of decision making within the practice, however the GP may become at risk of professional isolation.

- Health centres are run by the local NHS trust or health authority, and often employ many different types of healthcare professionals to offer a wide variety of services. This allows GPs to be part of a large interdisciplinary team.

GPs can also choose between working in a rural or inner-city practice. Each come with their own challenges and rewards. For example, in a rural area the doctor may have to travel long distances to visit their patients, but may be compensated for this by pleasant scenery and less traffic. However, practising a long distance from a hospital may require the doctor to deal with more urgent cases themselves and to be on-call more frequently. Working in an inner city practice may result in a GP encountering a wider variety of health issues, but may also result in the GP having to overcome language barriers and attempt to meet the healthcare demands in socially deprived areas.

Increasing numbers of GPs are extending their general skills or acquiring new skills to become a GP with a special interest (abbreviated to GPwSI and pronounced 'gypsy'). They are GPs that have additional experience and training in a specific clinical area, who take referrals for the assessment and treatment of patients that would otherwise have been directly referred to a hospital Consultant. The introduction of the GPwSI programme recognised the specialist skills that already existed in primary care, and allows GPs to help address the growing challenge of managing chronic disease in the community. Examples of interests that can be developed include drug misuse, family planning and women's health.

Becoming a GP

On nearing completion of the Foundation Programme, a doctor who aspires to become a GP will apply for entry onto the General Practitioner Vocational Training Scheme. At present, the specialty training for general practice is a minimum of three years; therefore the total time in training is five years following graduation. The three-year programme typically involves a series of placements with at least 12 months in general practice and around 24 months in a hospital setting. The programme is based on the Royal College of General Practitioners (RCGP) training curriculum approved by the PMETB. The aim of the curriculum is to address the wide knowledge base, professional attitudes and competences that are considered to be appropriate for a doctor practising in the NHS.

In order to be awarded their CCT doctors must succeed in passing the new RCGP examination. This consists of three elements, which include assessment of relevant knowledge, clinical skills, and a workplace based assessment. Upon successful completion of specialty training, doctors are placed on the GP register and become members of the RCGP.

Consultancy

After successful completion of medical school, the Foundation Programme and hospital based specialty training, a doctor can finally apply for a Consultant post. Since the introduction of MMC, the minimum length of training to become a Consultant is nine years from finishing medical school. The transition from specialty doctor to Consultant produces a variety of new pressures, challenges and complexities. The job of a Consultant is to act as a senior doctor, responsible for their own case load, as well as additional administrative and management tasks. Consultants provide qualified medical care for patients while leading a team (otherwise known as a firm), that comprises Specialty Registrars, doctors in their first years of specialty training, and foundation doctors.

After working for many years to reach this stage, doctors must be sure that the post they have selected is the right choice for them. An initiative called the New Consultant Entry Scheme was established to allow trusts and new CCT holders to 'sample' Consultant appointments for a six month period, giving CCT holders an opportunity to explore the Consultant role and learn more out about their employer without making immediate long term commitment. The scheme provides a sound basis for securing a permanent Consultant post if the doctor performs the temporary post successfully.

The role of the Consultant varies considerably across different specialties, as well as according to experience and seniority. For most Consultants, the main component of their role is formed by

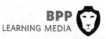

clinical responsibilities, which may include emergency duties, ward rounds, operating sessions, diagnostic work, out-patient clinics, multi-disciplinary team meetings and administrative care (such as patient referrals). Furthermore, all Consultants are involved in the teaching and education of medical students and junior doctors, which can take a variety of forms from bedside teaching to formal lectures. The role of teaching is essential in maintaining and improving standards of care for patients. In addition, many Consultants undertake research within the NHS as part of their own personal development, sustaining their own enthusiasm as well as making a valuable contribution to their field.

Becoming a Consultant

In order to become a Consultant, a suitable vacancy must become available. The trust that holds the vacancy will prepare a job description and a person specification for the post, and subsequently place an advertisement in relevant medical journals and publications. Applicants for the post will present themselves to an Advisory Appointments Committee, who conduct the interview process. Following the interview process, the Advisory Appointment Committee submit the name of the candidate deemed the most suitable to the trust board and employing authority. Once a post is offered, the doctor must agree a contract with their employer, and determine a job plan and work programme.

Until recently, there was little scope for flexible working, especially at Consultant level. However, the Improving Working Lives initiative has resulted in NHS employers increasingly developing more flexible ways for doctors to work and train. To some degree, Consultants are now able to shape their work to fit around their responsibilities, such as family and childcare. This is achieved through an arrangement with either the employer or the Flexible Careers Scheme. Arrangements can include job sharing (whereby two Consultants share one post), flexible working across a department with several Consultants covering the clinical workload, or part-time Consultant posts designed to alleviate the pressure from full-time colleagues. The Flexible Concert Scheme increases the scope for doctors to be able to work part-time and to return from career breaks.

Academic Medicine

Academic Medicine provides a pathway for doctors who wish to pursue a career in research, or to combine research with their clinical practice. Most academics maintain a specialist clinical practice while performing research, and / or providing teaching and training to undergraduates and postgraduates in Medicine and other associated professions. During the course of their training, doctors need to gain the necessary academic and clinical qualifications in order to pursue this career pathway. The UK Clinical Research Collaboration and MMC have established a training pathway for clinical academics to help establish the UK as a leader in the field of medical research.

Becoming an Academic Clinician

Medical students that are interested in pursuing a career in academic Medicine are advised to gain early research experience, for example via an Intercalated Bachelor Degree or MB PhD Programme (which incorporates a PhD within a medical degree). Furthermore, there are now Academic Foundation Programmes that have been specifically designed for doctors aiming to pursue a career in academic Medicine. The UKFPO estimates that around 5% of graduating medical students will apply to the Academic Programme. The necessary training is provided, as well as opportunities for training in research skills. As well as meeting the same clinical competencies as their colleagues on the standard Foundation Programme, individuals have time dedicated towards research in the second year of the programme. With the additional requirements, this is arguably a more challenging option, however for those interested in teaching and research well worth the additional effort. Places on the Academic Foundation Programme are limited and therefore competition for places can be very competitive.

Following the Foundation Programme, an academic training pathway is now in place that runs parallel to the standard clinical career pathway. This consists of three phases: Academic Clinical Fellowships, Clinical Lectureships and Clinical Senior Lectureships, which are equivalent to basic specialty training, higher specialty training and Consultant level posts, respectively.

Doctors that complete the Foundation Programme can apply for Academic Clinical Fellowships, along with doctors who are part

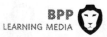

way through their specialty training. These posts are designed for doctors in the early years of their specialty training, and provide an environment for clinical and academic training. They are also designed for doctors preparing an application for a training fellowship in order to obtain a higher degree, or postdoctoral fellowship.

Clinical Lectureship posts are designed for doctors who already have experience in specialty training, or who hold a PhD / MD. The post provides teaching opportunities for doctors who are working towards the completion of their speciality training, or for research after obtaining a higher degree. The award of a Clinical Senior Lectureship aims to accommodate the new generation of Consultant level clinical academics who emerge from the Academic Clinical Fellowship and Clinical Lectureship training programmes.

Opportunities for GPs to join Academic Units are also being provided. There are Academic Clinical Fellowships that combine academic training with GP training, allowing GP trainees to set aside time in order to develop their academic skills, prepare their application for a training fellowship, and complete the GP scheme. GPs who are fully qualified and who already hold a higher degree are eligible to apply for Clinical Lectureships.

Other careers in Medicine

Despite the huge number of specialties and career pathways that are available within the NHS, some doctors opt for careers in other areas. As with particular specialties in Medicine and Surgery, there is a long list of options available, however, below are some common alternatives.

Specialty doctors

This is a specialist post for doctors with a minimum of four years postgraduate training (with two years in a relevant specialty). The role was designed for those who have been unable to progress through the normal training pathway; are from other countries; have been unable to gain a training post; failed to pass fellowship exams or assessments; or simply those who would prefer more regular working hours. As these doctors are not in training, their roles are more comparable to that of a Consultant. They focus more on NHS service provision and less on administration, and have less on-call responsibility, resulting in a more balanced lifestyle. It is important to note that specialty doctors are not at Consultant level as they have not completed the full training that is required.

Oral and maxillofacial surgery

This is a surgical specialty associated with diagnosis and treatment of disorders and diseases of the face, mouth, jaw and neck. This area of Medicine is unique and is mentioned separately in this section as it has specific entry requirements. In order to pursue this as a career you must have a degree in both Dentistry and Medicine. The majority of maxillofacial surgeons in the UK qualify in Dentistry before they qualify in Medicine, although there are a rising number of doctors in accelerated dental degrees, resulting in more medics achieving dual training. The specialist training after completion of both degrees lasts for five years, and upon successful completion of the examination and assessments, the specialist registrar will be awarded their CCT and will be eligible for appointment as a Consultant in oral and maxillofacial surgery. This branch of surgery will allow surgeons to work with all ages of patient, either in elective or emergency surgery. They frequently work alongside many other specialties including oncologists, neurosurgeons, orthodontists, plastic surgeons and ear, nose and throat surgeons.

Working in developing countries

This type of work tends to be in providing emergency relief, running clinical and medical education programmes and development work in building medical infrastructures. This offers the opportunity to gain valuable experience in some extremely challenging environments. It is preferable for doctors to have undertaken some specialty training, with the particularly useful specialties being Paediatrics, General Practice, Trauma and Surgery, and Obstetrics and Gynaecology.

The Armed Forces

There are many specialist roles available for both military and civilian doctors as an employee to the Defence Medical Services (DMS). Joining the DMS does not necessarily mean a long-term

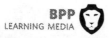

commitment with many doctors taking time out of their normal work to provide their services for a short period of time.

Prison health service

The majority of the work in this area is in primary care and prevention, although there is also a requirement for doctors with experience in communicable disease, mental health and drug abuse. Some specialty rotations require doctors to work within prison healthcare, and there are some part-time and full-time roles available.

There are many other career alternatives to the ones above, including Aviation Medicine, Expedition Medicine, Medical Law, Medical Journalism, Medical Politics and Medical Managers. A comprehensive list with a brief description of each can be found on the NHS medical careers website.

Doctors do have the opportunity to change specialty, however it is important to recognise that you must be able to meet the relevant competences required. The skills and knowledge that you will acquire in your training and day job could provide valuable resources to each of the jobs above, as well as furthering your development as a doctor.

 Summary

- There are many opportunities in Medicine, with a range of pathways available to allow doctors to reach their long-term goal.
- Medicine is constantly evolving. Some of the pathways that you read about now may have changed by the time you apply for your first job – it is wise to keep up to date with changes in the medical field.
- It is never too early to start thinking about a career pathway, however all doctors must be prepared for change and the fact that a career pathway might not go as planned.
- As you progress along your medical career make the most of all opportunities that arise.
- Gain as much experience as you can in a wide range of specialities.

- All experiences, good or bad, will contribute to your development as a doctor.
- Medicine is a highly rewarding career but is also one that requires commitment and a strong work ethic, so ensure that your chosen career path matches your own aspirations, as well as the needs of the health services.

 Useful resources

www.medicalcareers.nhs.uk
www.mmc.nhs.uk
www.foundationprogramme.nhs.uk
www.gmc-uk.org
www.nhscareers.nhs.uk
www.isfp.org.uk

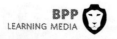

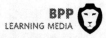

Chapter 10
Financial concerns

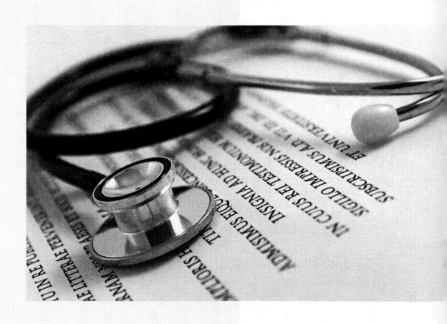

Financial concerns

If you are considering Graduate Entry Medicine, you will almost certainly have experienced three or more years at university already. Although you are now probably quite adept at dealing with the financial considerations that students face on a daily basis, there is a reasonable chance you will have incurred considerable debt during your first degree. For this reason, it is important that you are aware how much Graduate Entry Medicine is likely to cost.

Although a career in Medicine has the potential to be lucrative, this is usually not the case until many years in the future. Funding a Graduate Entry Medicine degree can appear complex and you will undoubtedly have many questions, such as: can I get a student loan? What is the NHS bursary? Are there any other sources of financial support? These questions have become even more pertinent with the rise in tuition fees for students starting in 2012.

This chapter aims to offer clear and uncomplicated answers to some of the common financial questions, allowing you to decide whether your investment is worthwhile or, indeed, feasible. The first half of the chapter outlines the major costs you are likely to incur, while the second half of the chapter discusses the major sources of funding. The chapter concludes by describing what you can expect to earn once you begin working as a doctor.

Expenditure

There are a number of costs associated with studying Graduate Entry Medicine before you have even commenced the course. While certain expenditures may be obvious, such as food and accommodation, many others which are not immediately apparent can quickly accumulate, such as buying smart clothes to wear at clinical placements. The following is a list of common expenses made by medical students on the graduate course.

Entrance exams

The first expense you are likely to incur when applying for Graduate Entry Medicine is the entrance exam fees. These vary depending on which tests you take and at what time in the year, as a higher cost is incurred if you register late for the UKCAT or BMAT. For

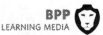

more information about entrance exams, please refer to Chapter 5. The following are the costs of taking the exams in 2011 for entry in 2012 and are likely to vary each year:

- UKCAT – £60 to £80 (£100 non-EU students)
- BMAT – £42.50 (£72.50 for non-EU students)
- GAMSAT – £195

Some students find it useful to invest in preparation material for these exams. There are a large selection of courses, books and online resources that provide advice and practice questions, the costs of which vary greatly. Whether or not you decide to pay for these resources is an individual decision. However, it is recommended that as a minimum you visit the website of the exam you will be taking early on to help familiarise yourself with the format of the tests. Other costs associated with applying to medical school include the UCAS application fee, Oxford and Cambridge application costs, and travel costs to attend open days and interviews.

Tuition fees

In line with the new funding arrangements for all students beginning higher education, there will be a significant rise in the tuition fees for students commencing Graduate Entry Medicine in 2012. The maximum tuition fee chargeable per year is £9,000. Most, if not all medical schools will charge this amount. To facilitate students during their studies, the Department of Health has agreed a new package of support for home students starting Graduate Entry Medicine from autumn 2012. This includes graduate entry students only having to self-fund the first £3,375 of tuition costs upfront in year one, payable either in full, or in instalments throughout the year. A student loan will be available for the remaining tuition fee. For the remaining years, tuition fees will be covered by a combination of a student loan and the NHS bursary. For further details on support available, please refer to the section in this chapter on income.

If you are classified as an international student, tuition fees are considerably higher. Applicants to 2012 entry can expect to pay between £13,400 and £18,400 per year during the pre-clinical years of the course and between £19,800 and £24,500 during the clinical years (figures based on 2009/2010 data).

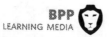

Travel costs

During the clinical years of medical school the majority of your time will be spent at placements in hospitals and GP surgeries. If you are eligible for an NHS bursary then you can reclaim the cost of travel and parking. If not, you will be expected to cover these costs yourself, although for distant placements a contribution towards travel may be available from your medical school. In some trusts you will also be required to pay for parking, the cost of which will vary considerably depending on location.

Course materials

You should expect to spend some money on course necessities. During the pre-clinical phase this will mainly involve the purchasing of books. Medical school libraries usually purchase multiple copies of the popular titles; however, most students choose to invest in at least two to three books on core topics such as anatomy, physiology and clinical medicine. You can expect to pay anything in the region of £20 to £60 for a standard textbook; however secondhand copies can often be bought from students in older years, medical libraries or online. During clinical placements you will be expected to purchase your own stethoscope, which will cost approximately £50. You will almost certainly need to invest in smart clothing for hospital and GP placements. Finally, as you near the end of your degree and medical school final exams approach, many students decide to take a revision course to assist them with the exam.

Medical elective

At some stage during the clinical years of the course, all medical students undergo a placement at a location and in a specialty of their choice. Many students use this as an opportunity to travel abroad and experience healthcare in a different environment. If you want to visit overseas, there are some bursaries available to help with elective costs; however, these are highly competitive so it is advisable to assume that these funds will not be available when budgeting for the placement. Alternatively, you may choose to spend your elective in the UK, which can be a good option if funds are limited. This provides an equally valuable opportunity for you to gain clinical experience in a hospital, or in a speciality you are particularly interested in.

Living costs

If you are considering applying to a Graduate Entry Medicine course then you will probably be familiar with the living costs associated with being a student, such as accommodation, travel and food. However, living costs vary greatly between locations, therefore it is advisable that you research the area you are considering moving to so you can avoid any financial shocks. Most universities provide an estimate of average living costs and these can usually be found on the finance pages of the respective university website. There is much to consider when predicting how much studying Graduate Entry Medicine will cost, but a few hours of careful planning will be worthwhile to avoid running into financial difficulties.

Income

There are a number of sources of funding available to Graduate Entry Medicine students. Most students rely upon several resources, due to the limited funds available from each individual source and the substantial costs associated with studying on the course. The following are a list of common resources available to most students.

Student loan

Having completed an undergraduate degree, you will most likely be very familiar with the student loan. Briefly, these are government loans administered by Student Finance England (formerly called the Student Loans Company). There is also Student Finance Wales, Student Finance Northern Ireland and Student Awards Agency for Scotland. Loans are available for maintenance and tuition fees.

Maintenance loans are available from years one to four and are calculated on a means-tested basis which takes parental earnings into account if you are classified as a dependent student, or personal earnings if you are classified as an independent student. In the first year only, you are eligible for a full means-tested maintenance loan of up to:

- £4,375 if you live with your parents.
- £5,500 if you are a non-London resident living away from home.
- £7,675 if you are a London resident living away from home.

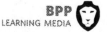

All eligible students will receive approximately 75% of the maximum loan, with the remaining amount calculated on a means-tested basis. This figure is dependent on your particular circumstances and is correct at the time of writing for the 2011/2012 academic year. From year two onwards, maximum student loans towards maintenance are reduced.

Tuition fees loans are available from years one to four and are not means-tested. In all years they are available to cover tuition fees, excluding the first £3,375. This remaining amount is payable by the student in year one or the NHS Bursary in years two, three and four (see below). Loan repayments do not start until the following April after you have either completed or left the course. Student Finance arrange repayments and automatically deduct 9% of any income earned in excess of £21,000 per annum. Comprehensive details on student loans for tuition fees and maintenance can be found at the government website, under the Education and Learning section.

You will apply for this loan in the same way as you would for a maintenance loan. If you are not familiar with this process, details can be found online at the student finance website. Applying for a student loan requires you to complete an application form, providing details of your course, living arrangements and parental income (if applicable).

NHS bursary

In years two, three and four of the graduate entry course you will receive support in the form of an NHS bursary, provided you meet the eligibility criteria (details of this are available on the NHS bursary website). This support will cover up to £3,375 of the tuition fee and is paid directly to the university. The NHS bursary can also provide financial support towards maintenance, consisting of a monthly sum paid directly into your bank account which does not need to be repaid. However, this bursary towards maintenance is 100% means-tested according to a variety of factors, such as your location, course length and parental earnings, or your own earnings if you have independent student status.

If you are a dependent student whose parental income totals less than £23,000 per year and you are living away from home in a non-London area, you can expect to receive in the region of £2,800 a year for a 30-week course. An additional non-repayable sum of around £80 is also provided for every extra week of the course beyond 30 weeks (which may be significant in the latter years of the course). The amount of bursary you are eligible for reduces if the amount of parental earnings increase, up to approximately £60,000, beyond which you will receive little, if any bursary.

Your university will liaise with the NHS bursary administration and a personal identification number will be generated which will be required for your application. You should note that the application for the NHS bursary is more detailed than for the student loan; it requires a number of original documents to be supplied by you and anyone supporting you. Therefore, it is recommended that you begin completing the form at the earliest opportunity to ensure your first payment arrives on time. More information on the NHS bursary, including the eligibility criteria and a 'Bursary Calculator' (that estimates the amount you are likely to receive), can be found on the NHS bursary website.

In years two, three and four, you can also reclaim the costs associated with travel to clinical placements. To receive this reimbursement from the NHS you will need to provide evidence of the expenditure incurred, for example, in the form of train tickets or bus receipts. If you drive and wish to claim for petrol then you will need to provide evidence that you are the owner of the car by submitting documents to verify your vehicle, such as a driving licence or insurance documents. Claims for travel costs are usually made via the university.

Please note that if you are a graduate on a five-year undergraduate medical degree, you would only be eligible for the above NHS support in your final year of study. This means you will have to pay tuition fees for all preceding years and you will also not be eligible for an NHS bursary, travel reimbursement or tuition fees loan. However, you will be eligible for a maintenance loan over this period. This is one of the major differences between the two courses and is an important consideration for those considering applying to the undergraduate course.

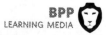

University grants, bursaries and scholarships

Many universities have funds available to support students from lower income families; therefore, it is worth checking with the medical school regarding additional support available. The conditions for eligibility can vary widely between universities so you are advised to enquire directly to the finance office once you know where you are likely to be studying. For example, the University of Birmingham awards medical students £860 per year if their parental income falls below a certain threshold. University bursaries are often only payable during the years in which NHS bursary support is not available

In the majority of cases, you will not need to complete additional applications to apply for such grants because the relevant information, such as household income, is passed directly from Student Finance to your university. For this information to be disclosed you will normally be required to indicate your consent by ticking the appropriate box on the online student loan application form. Occasionally, some universities will handle their own bursary schemes so it is important to check the policy of the university that you are considering applying to. Although often highly competitive, bursaries from a charitable organisation are available. There are many charities to which you can apply, each with their own eligibility criteria.

Professional/career development loans

Career development bank loans are available in amounts varying between £300 and £10,000. You can apply for a loan to help with tuition fees, living costs or any other expenses related to your course. They differ from ordinary commercial loans in that the Young People's Learning Agency pays the interest for the duration of your course and for one month afterwards. Interest rates vary, but as of June 2011 a career development loan can be taken out with an annual percentage rate of between 5 to 10%.

Some banks offer Professional Trainee Loans which are aimed at students training for certain professions, such as Medicine. These are available in amounts up to £20,000 and, as with career development loans, repayments do not take place until completion of the course. All bank loans will be subject to you meeting the bank's own eligibility criteria.

Part-time and summer work

You may consider whether it is possible to fund a Graduate Entry Medicine degree through part-time employment. There is no definitive answer to this question. A number of students inevitably take up part-time employment during evenings or weekends, and sometimes qualifications earned prior to starting Graduate Entry Medicine can enable students to earn enough to help support themselves. An example of this would be working as a locum pharmacist. Furthermore, skills and qualifications achieved during medical school can lend themselves to gaining part-time work, for example working as a first aider (after completing basic life support training).

However, Graduate Entry Medicine is not easy, and you should think carefully about whether you can cope with the additional workload and how this might affect your studies. If you are considering relying on part-time employment to supplement your income, it is advisable to speak to current students on the course to get an idea of whether this is feasible. You may find that part-time work is not recommended during certain phases of the course, but may be practical at other times.

Work during the summer holidays may also be possible. It might also be viable to secure a job related to Medicine, which could not only help with your finances but also add to your clinical experience, such as working as a healthcare assistant or in clinical research. However, it should be noted that the length of the summer holidays becomes progressively shorter as you advance through the course, making it increasingly difficult to work for substantial periods during the holidays.

Access to Learning Fund

Once you have begun your course, if you run into financial difficulties you may be eligible for support from your university's Access to Learning Fund which is designed to help students in hardship. Students studying Graduate Entry Medicine are eligible to apply via the university student services. The university will look at your individual circumstances before deciding whether to award you with any extra funding; you may need to provide evidence of financial hardship, such as bank statements, or bills

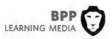

for this. Typical reasons for applying include unforeseen living costs, childcare, emergency payments for bills and (crucially) if you are thinking of leaving your course due to financial reasons. Any award is usually paid as a grant that does not have to be repaid, but the university can also decide to provide students with a loan depending on their circumstances.

Students with children

If you have children who are financially dependent on you then you are entitled to additional support. The two major sources of support are the Childcare Grant and the Parents Learning Allowance. The Childcare Grant can cover up to 85% of childcare costs up to a maximum of £148.75 per week for one child and £255 per week for two, or more children. The Parents' Learning Allowance pays between £50 and £1,508 depending on household income. Neither award requires repayment and you can apply for them via the standard student loan application form.

The Armed Forces

If you are considering a medical career with the Armed Forces (that is, the Army, Air Force or Navy) then funding arrangements can be quite different. You can apply for a medical cadetship while at university, which provides financial support during your medical degree. If you are successful in applying, from year two onwards you will be paid a salary of around £14,000 to £17,000 a year, in addition to having your tuition fees paid and receiving a textbook allowance of £150. However, in return you would be required to work for the Armed Forces as a medical officer for at least five years after Foundation Year 2. Further information can be found on the army website.

Doctors' salaries

Embarking on another degree is a considerable financial investment. So how long will it take to earn back this initial cost? The following outlines doctors' salaries as of 1 April 2011.

Doctors working in the NHS are paid a basic salary which is then supplemented, depending on contract hours. This is also known as banding. The basic salary paid to junior doctors at Foundation Year 1 level is £22,412 per year, rising to £27,798 in Foundation

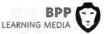

Year 2. The basic salary for doctors in speciality training starts at £29,705. The supplementary wage varies depending on the intensity of the post, but will usually be between 20% and 50% of the basic salary.

Doctors appointed at the speciality doctor grade will receive a basic salary of between £36,807 and £70,126, depending on experience and level of the post. The basic salary of a consultant working in the NHS is between £74,504 and £100,446 and can be supplemented by meeting certain target-based criteria. Finally, salaried general practitioners earn between £53,781 and £81,158, however many will be self-employed partners whose income will be dependent on meeting service criteria. Opportunities for private practice vary between specialties and will generally provide higher salaries.

Summary

- You can expect several major sources of expenditure from a medical degree, including:
  - Tuition fees
  - Living costs
  - Travel costs for placements
  - Course materials
  - Medical electives.
- To offset these costs, major sources of income include:
  - Student loans
  - NHS bursaries
  - University grants
  - Bursaries and scholarships
  - Professional/career development loans
  - Access to Learning Funds
  - Part-time/summer work.
- Financing another degree raises many issues but a few hours of careful planning will be very worthwhile to avoid encountering financial difficulties.
- Four more years of student life is a daunting prospect. However, if you are sure that Medicine is what you want to do, then there are various ways in which the costs can be covered – in which case, the ensuing investment could be viewed as the first step on the path to an enjoyable and potentially financially rewarding career.

Useful resources
www.nhscareers.nhs.uk
www.studentfinance.direct.gov.uk
www.money4medstudents.org
www.bursarymap.direct.gov.uk
www.ppa.org.uk/StudentBursariesCalculator/reset.do
www.army.mod.uk/join/join.aspx

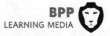

Chapter 11

Coping as a mature student

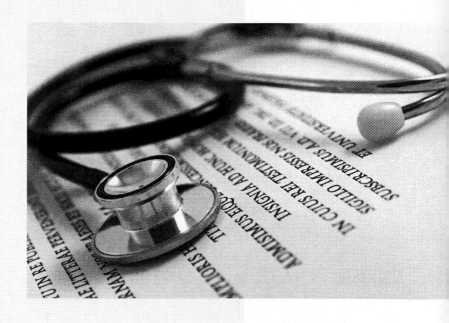

Coping as a mature student

The decision to study Medicine is a difficult one, and is potentially even more challenging for those considering Graduate Entry Medicine. If you are considering graduate entry, you will almost certainly be aged over twenty-one at the start of the course, and therefore be classed as a mature student. Being older than a typical medical student you are likely to have different considerations compared to a school or college leaver. For example, you may have spent time away from studying and therefore feel that you need to refine your study skills. Furthermore, having already completed one degree, and potentially having initially pursued a different career path, your time is limited compared to younger applicants, placing greater pressure on you to make the right decision.

As an older applicant, you may have commitments such as a house, partner or family which will need to be balanced with your studying commitments. Furthermore, having already paid for one degree, or having amounted debts from previous student loans, you may have more financial concerns than an undergraduate, and may need to work part-time to support your studies. Due to these additional considerations, much soul searching is required to answer questions such as, 'can I cope with being a student again?' or 'how will I manage with a family?' This chapter discusses the issues you may encounter returning as a mature student, such as balancing Medicine and working part-time, or having a family, as well as outlining ways that you can make the transition to returning to student life again as smooth as possible.

Returning as a graduate student

The possible routes you may have taken to commence a Graduate Entry Medicine course are extremely variable. For example, you may not have obtained the A level grades required for undergraduate Medicine and decided to pursue Medicine as a graduate, or you may have decided part-way through your first degree that you wanted to study Medicine. Alternatively, you may not have considered Medicine until after completing your first degree, after possibly commencing another career path.

Whatever route you have taken to commence a Graduate Entry course, you will have gained valuable experience that will advantage

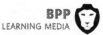

you along the way. For example, if you are proceeding from a recently completed degree you will have an abundance of newly acquired knowledge which, depending on the degree, could be very useful. In addition, you will be accustomed to study, revision and student life which may make settling into university life again easier.

There are also advantages if you have had some time off between degrees, as completing any degree is exhausting and therefore a period away from study can be refreshing and reinvigorating. Furthermore, a break between degrees can be a great opportunity to save money, gain relevant work experience, and even take the opportunity to travel. While there are many advantages to returning as a graduate to study Medicine, you will nevertheless face challenges along the way. The next section addresses some of these and suggests ways in which you may be able to deal with them effectively.

Coping with being a student again

Being accepted into medical school is a dream for many students, especially for graduate entry students where competition is that much more intense, but this does not necessarily mean that you will be psychologically ready to commence studying again. As a graduate, there are benefits and drawbacks to recommencing studying. For example, as a graduate student you will have spent at least three years studying for your first degree, and this additional academic (and life) experience can lead to many advantages over your undergraduate colleagues. This benefit is often most visible on the wards where, in general, graduates appear more calm and confident, particularly when things go awry.

However, being an experienced student can have its disadvantages, with some graduate students placing excess pressure on themselves. This often stems from graduate students having been proficient (and often excelling) in their previous field, to beginning Medicine where it can appear that everybody else knows more and is working harder. If you have these concerns, it is important to remember that pursuing a medical degree is a marathon, not a sprint, so pacing yourself and keeping perspective are vital skills, which as a graduate, you most likely already possess.

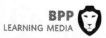

There are also certain skills which are vital to succeeding on the course, which as a graduate you should already have developed. These include learning effectively, being organised and having extra-curricular interests; these skills will be discussed in greater detail in the next section.

Studying

To become a doctor, medical students must devote four or more years to study how to diagnose and treat patients without accidentally doing them harm. Even when fully qualified, it is important to realise that you will be expected to keep up to date with current trends and practices. Although you will have completed a previous degree, your study skills may have lapsed, or you may find the demands of studying a graduate entry course more challenging. Therefore, before commencing the course you should review your approach to learning to ensure you will be able to study effectively.

Remaining alert and focused when you are studying is crucial and will be assisted by eating healthily, getting sufficient rest and avoiding too much caffeine and alcohol (an ideal not always achieved by students!). Although it is tempting, do not just sit down and start revising; you will retain much more information if you follow a structured approach, such as the one below:

- Make a study plan and decide which topics you will cover at the start of each session.
- Revise for about 30 to 45 minutes at a time and then take a short break.
- At the end of the session, examine yourself on the information covered by practising sample exam questions.
- Explain the topic to another person.

Organisation

Organisation is another aspect that can make a noticeable difference to a student's life. Indeed, this skill comes naturally to a fortunate few, however there are some easy ways that you can become more organised. One quick way to improve your organisation skills is to use a diary or wall planner to ensure that you always know where you need to be and when your deadlines are. This should enable you to plan your study time well in advance of deadlines and exam dates, to avoid having to 'cram' prior to exams, or having to rush to complete tasks near to deadlines. These approaches will undoubtedly help to reduce stress levels. Although some people work well under pressure, working into the night is not good for your health, or your concentration the following day! It may also help your organisation to keep notes in an ordered manner to make them easier to locate when you need them. In addition, note cards, post-its and highlighters can help to keep notes concise and emphasise key points. Finally, it is easier to be organised if you keep a dedicated study space, keeping notes and books where they are easy to locate and free of clutter.

Extra-curricular activities

As outlined in Chapter 6, taking part in extra-curricular activities prior to the application phase is important to demonstrate that you are a balanced individual. Such activities should not be abandoned once you have commenced the course, as maintaining a healthy lifestyle is crucial to coping at medical school. There is more to life than Medicine and sometimes acknowledging this can ease your mind and help you to retain perspective. Extra-curricular activities are an excellent way to reduce stress and increase energy levels as evidence suggests that two and a half hours of exercise per week can improve your physical and mental health, reduce your risk of some chronic diseases, increase self-esteem, and improve your quality of sleep.

In addition, demonstrating that you are able to undertake extra-curricular activities during your degree can be beneficial to your CV, which is important when applying for jobs as a doctor. You should endeavour to be active as much as possible, especially during stressful periods. There are many opportunities to participate in clubs and societies as a medical student, whereas once you are a junior doctor working long days, night shifts and weekends you may find it more difficult to maintain outside interests.

Communication skills

Your communication skills will greatly assist you while studying Graduate Entry Medicine, as much time will be spent talking and listing to other students, healthcare professionals, and patients. During the pre-clinical stage of Graduate Entry Medicine, almost

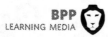

every course contains elements of PBL, where working as a group and being able to communicate effectively with others are key features. You will also be involved in other forms of group work, such as presentations, projects and reports throughout the course. As a graduate, you should have an advantage in this area, as you will almost certainly have worked in a group setting during your first degree or previous employment. This background will help you to make the most of these sessions which are a fundamental component of many graduate entry courses.

Furthermore, when starting clinical placements in hospitals or General Practices, you will need to appear confident and comfortable talking to patients and other healthcare professionals. This is more commonly observed in graduate entry students than their undergraduate colleagues. However, you should endeavour to further cultivate these skills throughout your time at medical school as they are fundamental once you are a qualified doctor, when it will be vital to develop a rapport with people. There are several ways that you can develop and improve your communication skills, such as:

- Maintain eye contact with the person you are speaking to.
- Use an appropriate tone and volume.
- Actively listen to the other person.
- Be aware of body language (such as having an open stance, facing the person and avoid crossing your arms).

Although keeping to your study schedule, being organised, maintaining a healthy lifestyle, and honing communication skills may seem like additional demands on your time, they will undoubtedly help you to cope with the pressures of being a student again. You may also find that as a mature student you have more commitments than a school leaver, such as a family, house or partner. Coping with these issues is discussed in detail below.

Balancing medical school and a family

As a mature student you are more likely to have, or to consider having a family during the course, compared to your undergraduate counterparts. Alternatively, you may have a long-term partner, and commencing another degree may involve you and your partner, or family, re-locating. Whether it is a long-term partner, children, or both, embarking on a Graduate Entry Medicine course will pose unique challenges to you and the other members of your family. Relationships involve compromise and sacrifice, and trying to find a happy equilibrium between family and a career may be difficult. Medicine can be an all-consuming lifestyle and sometimes it is difficult for non-medic partners to understand. Therefore it is vital that as a couple you both communicate with each other about how you are feeling.

If you are considering starting a family during your time at medical school, while it is not considered the norm, a growing number of graduate entry students have found themselves in this situation and have very successfully combined these two life-changing experiences. It must be acknowledged that having a family while being a student will certainly increase stress levels, however, how well you cope will depend on a variety of factors, including your previous life experiences, how much support you have available, and your financial security. Should you decide to start a family, there are some provisions available for time off from your studies, the length of this depending on whether you are an expecting mother or father.

Becoming a new mother during medical school involves significantly more challenges to overcome than becoming a new father. Medical schools are usually supportive and can accommodate students to their best abilities, but there are limits. If a student is unable to sit an exam and they have mitigating circumstances (giving birth is definitely one of these), they are usually offered to take the exam during the re-sit period, as if they were sitting the exam for the first time. If the same student is unable to take the re-sit exam then, in the majority of cases, they will have to wait until the next exam period the following year, before being able to progress. As a result, taking a year off the course is often the best option for a first-time mother. Another option is to have a shorter period of time off (three months is recommended for the health and wellbeing of mother and child) in which to give birth, and then attempt to catch up from where they stopped studying. How viable this option is will depend greatly on the university concerned and on which year of the course is affected.

Becoming a new father while at Medical School is a true test of how to cope under pressure, and male students should be aware

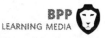

that depending on the delivery date, they may not be entitled to time off if it involves missing a compulsory part of the course. Aside from this, most medical schools will try to accommodate new fathers as much as they are able to and are likely to be able to offer in the region of two weeks off.

As mentioned in Chapter 10, graduate entry students may be eligible for an NHS bursary and with the birth of a new child these students may qualify for further grants from the NHS. Women who decide to take maternity leave from medical school and who are eligible for an NHS bursary can apply for the NHS maternity award. In addition, students with children who are cared for during the day by a childcare provider may be eligible for an allowance depending on their financial circumstances. Please check the NHS website for further details.

Working part-time as a Graduate Entry Medicine student

As a mature student, you may have amassed considerable debts or loans following your first degree, and there is often a temptation to work part-time to contribute towards the living costs of being a full-time student. While it is possible to undertake paid work part-time during a medical degree it is, nevertheless, challenging to maintain the right balance.

Should you decide to work part-time, graduate students are at a significant advantage over their undergraduate colleagues in securing work, having already gained a degree, and in many cases having already worked prior to commencing the course. For example, students who have a healthcare qualification such as pharmacy or midwifery may easily find work as a locum at weekends. However, you should bear in mind that jobs that require working late on weekdays, or even throughout the night are not very practical to prepare you for a day at university or in hospital. Holiday periods are an excellent opportunity to work, as they avoid taking up valuable study time, however, holidays on Medicine courses are generally shorter than for other degrees and therefore the amount of time available is somewhat restricted.

Whether it is a feasible to work during term time will also depend partly on the style of the course. For example, it may be more difficult in a PBL-style course where weekends are a good time to study further. Also, for graduate entry courses with an accelerated pre-clinical phase, it may be advisable to refrain from working during this part of the course, as the workload can be particularly heavy. However, once integrated onto the standard course, you are likely to have more free time (which would enable you to manage your time to include paid employment).

Although it is possible to work part-time while studying, bear in mind that working to earn money during a medical degree is generally not recommended by medical schools, as time spent working can be at the expense of fully covering the undergraduate curriculum. Furthermore, you will need to be extremely organised and focused to avoid falling behind your cohort and the risk of failing exams. If money is a serious issue, taking out a student or commercial loan may be an option to gain more financial flexibility during the course of the degree, while still allowing you the time to study or simply to relax.

 Summary

- Commencing a degree as a mature student will be challenging, especially given the demands of the Graduate Entry Medicine course.
- Returning to study may involve:
  - Difficult decisions
  - Close communication with family and partners
  - Extensive time management to ensure all your commitments are met.
- Ensure that you have seriously considered the advantages and disadvantages of becoming a student again and, most of all, of becoming a doctor.
- To make a truly informed decision, try to gain as much healthcare experience as possible to be certain that Medicine is the right career path for you. Should you decide that it is, the skills and experience that you will have acquired during your previous degree will assist you.
- Maintain a life outside of Medicine to relieve stress and enable you to keep a balanced perspective during difficult times.

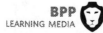

- Remain organised, and plan your time to study sufficiently, and meet deadlines.
- Working part-time is feasible; however it will take excellent time management skills to avoid over-committing yourself.
- There will be many demands on your time, but it is worth remembering that there is never a perfect time to have or raise a family. Having a family while being a student may offer more flexibility than at any other stage in your career.

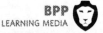

Chapter 12

After an unsuccessful UCAS application

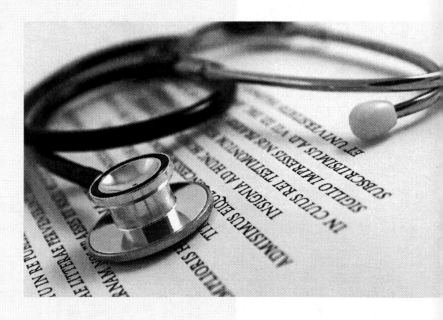

After an unsuccessful UCAS application

Inevitably, many applicants to Graduate Entry Medicine will be unsuccessful in their first time of applying due to the high levels of competition for places. This chapter will assist you in coping with a failed application, and will explore common reasons you may not have been successful, from the UCAS application form and entrance exam, to the interview. The chapter will then outline the options available to you, such as re-applying to Graduate Entry Medicine or applying to a different course. The chapter concludes with suggestions on ways to improve your application, should you decide to re-apply.

Coping with an unsuccessful application

This may be your first experience of academic failure and could potentially lead to lack of self-confidence and motivation. Indeed, you may even feel like giving up completely, however, by this stage you will have invested much time and thought in considering your future career path. Therefore it is important to avoid making any rash decisions. Failing to be given an offer, or not achieving the conditions set by a medical school, may mean a delay to your entry to medical school, or change in the medical school you attend, but does not necessarily mean you will not be able to study Medicine. In the event of an unsuccessful application, there are several useful strategies for coping, including:

- Accepting and adjusting to the reality of your unsuccessful application
- Maintaining a positive self-image
- Self-reflection
- Planning effectively to ensure future success
- Seeking social or emotional support

Importantly, instead of focusing on not receiving an offer, you should concentrate on what you are going to do next. You should seek feedback early on and use this constructively to decide on your course of action and the steps you will need to take to achieve this. It is vital that you reflect upon your feedback to identify possible weaknesses which could be improved for future applications. At the same time, you should avoid being overly critical of yourself;

instead, talk to friends or family about how you are feeling, and remember to keep in mind that Medicine is a very popular course and every year many strong applicants are unable to secure a place at one of their chosen medical schools. This is even more common in the case of Graduate Entry Medicine, where the ratio of applicants to places is generally higher. As a result, every year universities have to reject many candidates who would make excellent doctors due to the limited number of places they can offer.

Why was I unsuccessful?

After receiving a rejection from one of your four choices, regardless of which stage in the process this occurs, you will undoubtedly ask yourself why you were unsuccessful. Medical schools may or may not provide the rationale behind their decision on the tracking facility on the UCAS website. If you have not received any information via UCAS, it is advisable to contact the medical school directly to seek feedback on your application. Although medical schools are not obliged to offer feedback, many will happily do so.

There are many possible reasons that you may have been declined, such as a poorly written personal statement, lack of work experience, a weak interview, failure to achieve entrance exam requirements or failure to meet the conditions of your offer. It may simply be the case that as competition for places is high, your application was not as good as that of other applicants, despite you achieving the minimum requirements. After gaining feedback, the important thing is to take time to consider each area of weakness in turn and work towards improving them for subsequent applications.

Options available to unsuccessful candidates

Having adjusted to not being accepted to any of the medical schools you applied to, you will no doubt wonder what to do next. With the benefit of an additional year of preparation, it is possible to significantly improve your application by working on one or more aspects of your application, such as work experience, entry exams your personal statement or your interview technique.

At this stage, most unsuccessful university applicants are encouraged to apply through clearing to try to get onto their chosen course; however, it is important to note that Medicine courses are rarely

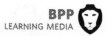

available through clearing, if at all, due to their popularity and the high levels of competition. Instead, there are three main options available to applicants who have been declined offers from all four medical schools they applied to:

- Apply to Undergraduate Medicine (or a combination of Undergraduate and Graduate Entry Medicine)
- Re-apply to Graduate Entry Medicine
- Apply to an alternative healthcare profession

Applying to undergraduate Medicine

If you decide to apply to an Undergraduate Medicine course it is important to check, prior to submitting an application, that the medical school accepts graduates onto the undergraduate course as medical schools vary considerably on their policy of accepting graduates (see the Appendix for a list of medical schools who accept graduates). Again, be aware that you will most likely need to take one or more entrance exams in the process. There are some advantages and disadvantages to applying to Undergraduate Medicine; one of the major benefits is that Undergraduate Medicine courses are generally less competitive and therefore your chances of being accepted are greater. However, a disadvantage of Undergraduate Medicine is the additional one to two years required to qualify (opposed to Graduate Entry Medicine). Another major drawback is the reduced funding available compared to Graduate Entry Medicine (for a more detailed comparison between Undergraduate and Graduate Entry Medicine, please refer to Chapter 3.). If you are considering applying to both undergraduate and graduate entry courses at a particular medical school, be sure to check that this is acceptable in advance, as some medical schools will not permit applicants to apply to both courses in the same academic year. Finally, remember that the total number of medical courses you can apply to is four, regardless of whether they are graduate entry or undergraduate courses.

Applying to an alternative healthcare profession

There are several options available which would still enable you to work within the caring professions, should you choose not to reapply to Medicine. These include applying to an alternative healthcare profession, such as a physician assistant, or one of the allied health professions, such as:

- Arts therapists
- Chiropodists
- Dieticians
- Occupational therapists
- Operating department practitioners
- Orthoptists
- Prosthetists
- Psychotherapists
- Radiographers
- Physiotherapists
- Psychologists
- Speech and language therapists

Some of these career paths have fast-track routes for graduates, for example, physicians assistant, psychologist, and speech and language therapist. For more information on the careers listed above, please refer to the NHS Careers website which now includes a dedicated section entitled 'what can I do with my degree?'

Physician assistant

A physician assistant is a healthcare professional who is qualified to practise Medicine under the direct supervision of a qualified doctor, supporting them in the management of patients. They provide a range of services that are traditionally performed by a physician including history-taking, examination and treatment. Similar to Graduate Entry Medicine, admission to the course requires a previous degree, usually in life sciences or a health-related discipline. Although the course has only been developed in the UK recently, it has been established for many years in the US. There are currently three universities running the Physician Assistant Diploma course in the UK:

- The University of Birmingham
- St. George's, University of London
- The University of Wolverhampton

All physician assistant courses are two years in duration; however, they differ considerably in structure, and the proportion of how much of the course is taught and how much is self-directed.

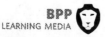

Standard tuition fees apply, and following successful completion of the course, salaries are in the region of £22,500 and £32,000. For more information, please visit the UK Association of Physician Assistants website or the university websites.

Clinical psychologist

A clinical psychologist is a healthcare professional who uses scientific methods to help people overcome mental health problems including depression, phobias, stress and addictions. It is one of several disciplines within Psychology including educational, forensic, and occupational Psychology.

Non-Psychology graduates may become eligible for Graduate Basis for Chartered Membership to the British Psychological Society by completing an accredited conversion course (graduate diploma). This takes one year full-time or two years part-time. Once attained, it is possible to apply for a paid training post which leads to registration with the Health Professions Council.

Applicants are expected to possess a good honours degree and good pass grades at A Level, and must be able to demonstrate an understanding of scientific concepts. Universities are often flexible regarding which A Levels are required, though some courses require 60 UCAS credits in undergraduate level Psychology studies (these can be achieved by completing an associate course, often run by the university itself as an 'Introduction to Psychology' over two or three modules, or part time study, or through the Open University 'Exploring Psychology' course). For more details of courses see the British Psychological Society website.

Speech and language therapist

Speech and language therapists (SLTs) are healthcare professionals who work with people to treat communication, speech and language problems. They work with people of all ages including children, and patients who suffer from a range of problems, including strokes, learning disabilities, neurological disorders, injuries, deafness, psychological disorders, and eating and swallowing problems. SLTs mainly work for the NHS, in hospitals, community health centres, schools, and day centres.

Entry requirements are a minimum of two or three good A Levels pass grades. With an appropriate first degree, applicants can take an accelerated two-year postgraduate qualification, leading to a postgraduate diploma or masters degree. Universities that offer the course are:

- Queen Margaret University, Edinburgh
- City University, London
- Canterbury Christ Church University
- The University of Greenwich

For more information please see the Royal Society of Speech and Language Therapists website.

Re-applying to Graduate Entry Medicine

If you decide to re-apply to Graduate Entry Medicine courses, there are some things to bear in mind. The first point to note is that if your application is unsuccessful one year, most universities will allow you to re-apply the following year without fear that your previous application will prejudice your new application. However, you must contact the respective university if you intend to reapply the following year, to ensure that they accept previous applicants.

It is also important to factor how long your entrance exam results are valid for, as GAMSAT results are currently valid for two years, whereas BMAT and UKCAT results are only valid for one year and therefore must be retaken if you are re-applying. However, there is no limit to the amount of times these entrance examinations may be sat. If you did not achieve the sufficient entrance exam result, or if you plan to retake an entrance test and you feel you did not prepare thoroughly first time around, plan well in advance to ensure you are as prepared as possible for the subsequent test. It is worthwhile to invest in a practice exam book or consider attending a course, as even a few additional correct answers can make a significant difference. See Chapter 9 for further information on entrance exams.

It is also important to carefully consider whether to apply to the same medical schools as your first application, or to apply elsewhere. You may decide to apply to less competitive medical

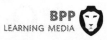

schools or those that use a different entrance exam. Alternatively, you may decide to apply to the same medical schools; however, this is only advisable if you feel you can submit a significantly stronger application the second time round. This decision-making process requires much thought as it is important to balance your preference of medical school against an assessment of where you are most likely to be accepted.

What to do next?

It is important to make the most of your time between applications. Remember that there are many options available, and by being proactive you should be able to find something which is both enjoyable and worthwhile. It is valuable to consider options that will improve your application and increase your chances of success, such as work experience or voluntary work. This may even include working overseas, for example in a school, hospital or a community project in a developing country. Such experiences can be highly rewarding and give you an alternative perspective to healthcare provisions, as well as being a great opportunity to travel and learn about a different culture. Alternatively, you may decide to use the year to gain research experience in an area related to Medicine.

Improving your application

If you have decided to re-apply to Graduate Entry Medicine, or to apply to Undergraduate Medicine, it is important to attempt to improve your application in a systematic way in order to maximise your chances of a successful application the following year. A useful approach is to consider the three main stages of the application process. For the majority of courses, these are: the entrance exam, the UCAS application and the interview. For each of these stages, several different attributes are assessed, from your qualifications and work experience, to your extra-curricular activities.

Remember that university applications are assessed, not only on the basis of academic achievements, but also by non-academic criteria by means of the personal statement and the interview. While it may be difficult to improve your academic background, improving your non-academic credentials is a feasible and reasonable way to enhance your application. Furthermore, most students who reach the interview stage of the application have already met the academic entry requirements; therefore, if you reached this stage of the application process it is advisable to focus on improving the non-academic aspects of your application. There are a range of ways you can improve your application for a subsequent reapplication. Some of the main ones are listed below.

Pre-interview stage

Entrance exams

Your application may have been unsuccessful due to your entrance exam marks not being sufficiently high enough, or you may feel that this area was relatively weak compared to other aspects of your applications – remember, even a small increase in your score can make the difference between being offered an interview or not. To perform well at entrance exams, you must become familiar with the format of questions and answering questions under timed conditions. Even the strongest of students benefits from knowing what to expect, understanding the specific question types used, and appreciating how to organise their time through the completion of multiple practice tests. Therefore, if you did not prepare thoroughly first time around, be sure to do so on your subsequent attempts by investing in the appropriate resources available. See Chapter 7 for more information on entrance exams.

UCAS statement

Your feedback may specifically refer to you not fully demonstrating the qualities required to become a doctor, or you might feel that this area of your application could be improved. You should therefore compare your previous application to the skills and qualities laid out in *Tomorrow's Doctors* (2009) to assess whether you have demonstrated these. To improve your application, ensure that you have included examples of when you have demonstrated all of these qualities, which may be as a result of additional work experience or extra-curricular activities that you have undertaken since your initial application. For example, you may decide to use the opportunity between applications to take up a new hobby or gain additional clinical experience which will make your application more interesting. Given the intensity of a medical career, admissions panels like to see candidates who are able to balance their work with outside interests to help them manage the challenges they are likely to encounter.

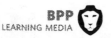

To further enhance your personal statement, it is advisable to have as many people as possible critique it to allow you to present your strongest possible application. For example, friends, family and medical professionals you are acquainted with may all be able to give you useful advice on improving your personal statement. Another option is to seek the advice of a careers advisor for a professional opinion, as they are likely to possess a great deal of experience in enhancing written applications.

Your feedback may have stated that you demonstrated insufficient work experience, or you may feel that you are lacking experience within the healthcare setting. In these cases it is advisable to attempt to gain additional experience in the time between applications in order to turn this area into a strength. Every medical school requires applicants to have gained some experience in a healthcare environment, such as a hospital or a residential home, and some medical schools even quantify the minimum amount required.

Long-term voluntary commitments and healthcare work significantly improve your application, provided they afford you with clinical experiences that you are able to learn from. For example, you may wish to get a job as a healthcare assistant or phlebotomist, both of which will give you highly useful clinical experience. Alternatively, you could spend time volunteering in a hospital, or a GP practice centre, either in the UK or abroad. Not only would this be a rewarding experience, but could also give you a new perspective on working as a healthcare profession. Furthermore, attaining work experience in more than one environment facilitates better reflection and a greater appreciation of healthcare provision in the UK and abroad.

Interview stage

In the event that you were unsuccessful after being invited for an interview, it is important to reflect upon your UCAS application in addition to the interview itself. Was it a single event that was responsible, or a combination of factors? As with entrance exams, the two major pitfalls at this stage are excessive nerves and insufficient preparation. When considering your performance at interview, you should review the types of questions that you were asked and whether you answered these fully, using appropriate examples.

To improve your responses, devise a model answer and compare this to the actual answer you gave during the interview.

The key to answering the majority of medical school questions is presenting a well-argued and structured answer, coupled with a calm and professional demeanour. For example, were your responses supported by pertinent and valuable experiences, or were there times when you attempted to fabricate answers? If so, remember that the interview panel are not looking to hear the same generic answers from every applicant but rather individually tailored responses that reflect your own personal experience. Reflect upon how the interview panel may have perceived you and attempt to address any weaknesses in your interview technique – preparation is unquestionably the key to succeeding at interviews.

An important area to consider is how you reacted to being questioned. Did you take time to think through your answers before responding, or did you rush to give an immediate answer? Were you able to explain your reasoning articulately, or did you struggle to make yourself clear? Did you answer all the questions you were asked, or did you instead answer the questions you had prepared answers to? If you could not answer a question, or realised that what you going down the wrong track, were you honest and acknowledge the mistake? If you did not, practise your response, should you be asked the question again.

If, on reflection you decide that your knowledge of medical issues was your weak area at interview, you have a year to rectify this. For example, if your answer to questions on medical controversies or the medical profession was vague, use this time to research these areas in detail, looking at notable articles in the media and keeping up with current medical affairs. When acquainting yourself with a new topic, practise discussing the area with someone else to become accustomed to the experience of being interviewed.

Alternatively, if you feel that your interview technique was your main problem, than you need to dedicate time to cultivate this skill. Again, the most useful way to improve your technique is to experience as many mock (or real) interviews as possible, coupled with feedback to identify your weaknesses. See Chapter 8 for further advice on interview technique.

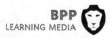

Post-interview stage

This applies to applicants who were successful at interview and received a conditional offer, but who were unable to meet the conditions of that offer. If you missed the grades required you will need to research whether this is a surmountable problem. For example, if you did not gain the degree classification required, is it possible to study for a particular module or a higher degree (such as a Masters) to circumvent the missed grade? If these are not options could you apply to the undergraduate course instead?

 Summary

- Being unsuccessful at gaining a place at medical school is a difficult scenario for anyone to experience, but it is extremely important to remember that this setback is not necessarily the end of your medical career and there are plenty of options available to you. You may choose to:
    - Apply to Undergraduate Medicine
    - Reapply to Graduate Entry Medicine, or
    - Change your application to an alternative or allied healthcare profession course.
- You should obtain feedback on your application from UCAS or from the medical schools themselves as early as possible, and use this feedback constructively to assess the strengths and weaknesses of your application.
- You should strive to improve your application, perhaps by:
    - Gaining more work experience
    - Improving the style or content of your personal statement
    - Taking on additional extra-curricular activities
    - Practising entrance exam questions, and
    - Undertaking mock interviews.
- Use this additional year to significantly improve your application to ensure you are successful in whatever area you decide to pursue the following year.

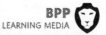

Appendix

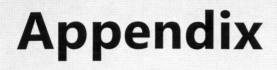

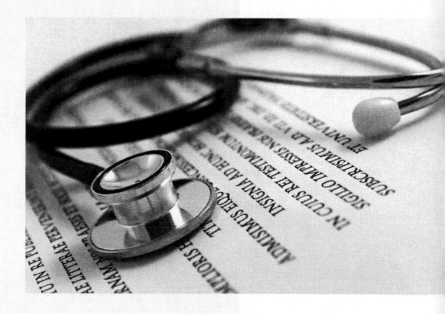

Appendix

Useful resources

- www.ucas.ac.uk/students/track
- www.nhscareers.nhs.uk
- www.whatcanidowithmydegree.nhs.uk/
- www.ukapa.co.uk (UK Association of Physician Assistants)
- www.wlv.ac.uk (University of Wolverhampton)
- www.birmingham.ac.uk (University of Birmingham)
- www.sgul.ac.uk (St George's, University, London)
- www.bps.org.uk (British Psychological Society)
- www.rcslt.org.uk (The Royal College of Speech and Language Therapists)
- www.qmu.ac.uk (Queen Margaret University, Edinburgh)
- www.city.ac.uk (City University, London)
- www.gre.ac.uk (University of Greenwich)
- www.canterbury.ac.uk (University of Canterbury)
- www.gapyear.com
- www.projects-abroad.co.uk/volunteer-projects/medicine-and-healthcare/electives
- www.gvi.co.uk (volunteer abroad)
- www.kaptest.co.uk/default.aspx
- www.medicalinterviewsuk.co.uk/medical-school-interviews/medical-students.html

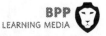

Five-year courses that accept graduates

A list of universities which offer five-year courses are stated below; for further details and entry requirements, please see the respective university website:

- University of Aberdeen
- Barts and The London School of Medicine and Dentistry
- University of Birmingham
- Brighton and Sussex Medical School
- University of Bristol
- University of Cambridge
- Cardiff University
- University of Dundee
- The University of Edinburgh
- University of Glasgow
- University of Hull
- Imperial College London
- Keele University
- King's College London
- University of Leeds
- University of Leicester
- University of Liverpool
- The University of Manchester
- Newcastle University
- The University of Nottingham
- University of East Anglia, Norwich Medical School
- University of Oxford
- University of Sheffield
- University of Southampton
- University of St Andrews
- University College London

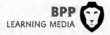

Glossary

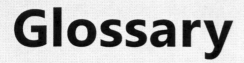

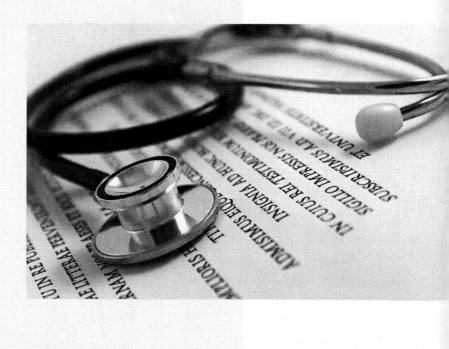

Glossary

Academic Foundation Programme – A two-year training programme for new doctors that provides opportunities to undertake research and teaching, in addition to having a clinical role as a doctor.

Accelerated degree – A full degree completed over a shortened period of time, such as Graduate Entry Medicine.

Admissions Officers – Staff who work in a University Admissions Office who are responsible for the processing of UCAS applications and organising the application process.

Allied health professions – An umbrella term used for healthcare workers who are not doctors, dentists or nurses, such as a paramedics and physiotherapists.

Autonomy – One of the four key principles underlying medical ethics. Refers to the capacity of a rational individual to have self-directing freedom and moral independence.

Bachelor's degree – A higher education qualification awarded for an undergraduate course, sometimes known as a 'first' degree.

Beneficence – One of the four key principles underlying medical ethics. Refers to acting in the best interest of others.

BMAT – Biomedical Aptitude Test. A selection test used by some Medical Schools as part of the application process.

Career break – A period of time spent out of employment, often for personal and/or professional development, travelling or to raise children.

Clearing – A process operated through UCAS, whereby applicants who have not been offered a place on a course through an initial application can apply to courses that have become available.

Clinical placement – A length of time during a medical degree spent in a hospital or General Practice.

 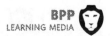

Clinical years – A stage during the course of a medical degree when placed all, or most of the time, in a clinical environment, such as a hospital or General Practice.

Clinicians – Another term for medical doctor who has direct contact with, and responsibility for patients.

Conditional offer – An offer made by a university or college through UCAS which is dependent on the applicant meeting some form of academic criteria.

CRB check – Check for current and spent convictions, cautions, reprimands and relevant information held by local police forces and the Police National Computer.

CV – Curriculum Vitae. A document which is typically sent to prospective employers when applying for a job, or accompanies an application form, summarising the applicant's educational qualifications and employment history.

Deaneries – Regional organisations within the NHS that are responsible for postgraduate medical and dental training.

Deferral – Delaying, or holding an offer until the following year.

Didactic – A traditional teaching style whereby a teacher imparts information to an audience.

Elective – A period of study during a medical degree, which is not part of the core curriculum, whereby students undertake a clinical placement or research project in an area of interest, either at their medical school or further afield.

Flexible working – A variable work schedule, allowing employees to work alternative hours to the standard working week.

Foundation Programme – A two-year structured programme of workplace-based learning, following the completion of medical

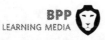

school, whereby newly qualified doctors are able to apply their knowledge, and train in a variety of different specialties.

Foundation schools – A junior doctor training school in the UK, providing training to junior doctors in a range of clinical settings to enable them to complete the Foundation programme.

GAMSAT – Graduate (Australian) Medicine Schools Admissions Test. A selection test used by some Medical Schools as part of the application process.

Gap year – A period of time, usually one academic year, that a student can choose to take before commencing college or university, often to gain work experience or to travel.

General Practice – Run by General Practioners, they provide primary un-specialised care and are often the first port-of-call for non-emergency problems, diagnosing and treating acute and chronic illnesses, and providing healthcare information to individuals, families and the community.

Group practices – A medical practice run by several doctors and medical professionals.

Health centres – A centre owned by a local authority, which provides healthcare for the community, usually via a medical practice, as well as providing other services such as child or X-ray services.

Healthcare assistant – Someone who works within a hospital or community, providing care to patients under supervision of a qualified health professional.

Home student – Students from the United Kingdom including Scotland, Northern Ireland and Wales, The Channel Islands, The Isle of Man and students from the European Union.

Honours degree – A degree course that requires a higher academic standard than a pass degree, although in England the majority of bachelor's degrees are now honours degrees.

Hospice – A type of care provided to a terminally ill person, including physical, psychological, social and spiritual support. Can be inpatient and outpatient care.

Insurance choice – A course selected by an applicant that they intend to take if they do not meet the academic requirements of their first choice.

Intercalated degree – An optional, additional year of study during a medical degree which involves studying an area of Medicine in greater depth leading to the award of a bachelor's degree.

Job sharing – An employment arrangement where one job is split between two or more employees, working on a part-time basis.

Justice – One of the four key principles underlying medical ethics. Refers to treating patients in a fair way.

Lay person – A person who is a non-expert in a given field of knowledge.

Maastricht seven step process – A structured model used in Problem-based learning which involves seven stages, developed at Maastricht University, Netherlands.

Masters degree – An academic degree available to graduates with a bachelor's degree awarded to individuals who have undergone advanced studies of a specific field of study.

MD – Literally meaning 'Teacher of Medicine', in the UK refers to an advanced academic research degree, known as a doctorate in Medicine.

Mind map – A diagram that centres around a key word or idea, around which other items are linked or arranged, used to generate ideas.

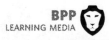

Multi Mini Interview system (MMI) – A structured interview system whereby candidates move between timed stations where they are interviewed and marked independently by interviewers.

NHS Bursary – A fund available to students on healthcare courses such as Medicine. Provides non-repayable support to assist with living costs and tuition fees during a course of study. Consists of income assessed and non-income assessed components.

NICE – National Institute for Health and Clinical Excellence. A body that provides guidance for doctors on best practices.

Non-maleficience – Derives from the Latin 'first, do no harm', and is an obligation avoid harm to a patient wherever possible.

On-call rotas – An arrangement that doctors provide 'out-of-hours' cover to patients.

PhD – The highest degree possible in a given field. It typically takes three years to complete, is normally purely research-based, and requires the candidate to submit a thesis.

Postdoctoral fellowship – Academic or scholarly research conducted by somebody who has completed medical studies, in order to develop expertise in a specialty.

Pre-clinical stage – The initial period of a medical degree which is spent predominantly at a university prior to undertaking placements in a clinical environment.

Primary care trust – A type of NHS trust that provides, or commissions some primary and community services, and is involved in commissioning secondary care.

Problem-based learning (PBL) – A student-centred approach to teaching in which students collaboratively solve problems and reflect on their experiences.

Prospectus – A publication from a university giving an overview of the university and courses offered.

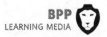

Royal Colleges – Medical professional societies responsible for the training of doctors within a different specialty of the medical field.

Run-through training – A type of training post, whereby once appointed, the trainees continue through to the completion of specialty training, provided all the required standards are met.

Scholarship – A financial grant or payment that supports a student's education, which is awarded on the basis of academic merit or another achievement.

Self-directed learning – A form of learning whereby students are responsible for their own learning, including setting priorities, identifying targets, organising study, and evaluating performance.

Shadowing – A form of work experience whereby you learn by observing a person doing a job.

UCAS – Universities and Colleges Admissions Service is a non-profit, non-government charitable organisation that is responsible for managing applications to almost all full-time undergraduate degree programmes at UK universities and colleges.

UKCAT – UK Clinical Aptitude Test. An entrance exam used by many Medical and Dentistry Schools as part of the application process.

Unconditional offer – An offer made by a university or college, whereby you have met all the academic requirements to be accepted on the relevant course.

Uncoupled training – Specialised training that is divided into two phases. Having completed the initial phase trainees must then compete to gain entry to the second part of specialty training.

Work experience – time spent doing a job in an ordinary work environment in order to gain experience of employment, usually unpaid.

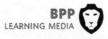

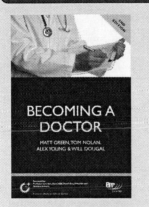

More titles in the Entry to Medical School Series

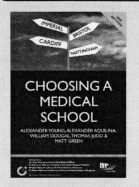

CHOOSING A MEDICAL SCHOOL

ALEXANDER YOUNG, ALEXANDER AQUILINA, WILLIAM DOUGAL, THOMAS JUDD & MATT GREEN

£19.99
November 2011
Paperback
978-1-445381-50-3

Choosing which Medical Schools to apply to is a decision that should not be taken lightly. It is important that you do your homework and consider carefully the many factors that differ between each institution.

This comprehensive and insightful guide written by medical students, for medical students, covers everything you need to know to enable you to select the Medical Schools best suited to you. The book is designed to help school leavers, graduates and mature individuals applying to Medical School, together with parents and teachers.

The first part of the book covers what to expect from life at medical school and things to consider prior to applying.

The second part then features chapters covering each individual UK Medical School. Each chapter is written by current medical students at the institution and is broken down into sections on the medical school, the university and the city finishing with the views of pre-clinical and clinical students.

This book is best used in conjunction with 'Becoming a Doctor'.

Key Features:

- **Forewords** - by Sir Liam Donaldson (Chief Medical Officer of England), Professor Ian Gilmore (President of Royal College of Physicians), Mr John Black (President of Royal College of Surgeons) and Professor Mike Larvin (Director of Education Royal College of Surgeons)

- **Insider Information** - An overview of what to expect from life at Medical School and tips for getting in and staying ahead

- **Latest Admission Statistics and Advice** - Up-to-date information on course structure, teaching methods, entrance requirements and other key factors to consider when choosing a Medical School

- **Pre-Medical and Postgraduate Advice** – views from preclinical and postgraduate students on getting in and what to consider

- **Easy Comparisons** - Quick comparison table covering each UK Medical School

- **Medical Education** - Clear sections focussing on pre-clinical and clinical education including summaries of teaching methods, support, examinations and teaching hospitals

- **Extracurricular Activities** - Information on what extracurricular opportunities are available at each Medical School and in the surrounding city

- **Students' Views** - Opinions and insights for each Medical School by current medical students

By using this engaging, easy to use and comprehensive guide, you will remove so much of the uncertainty surrounding how to best select the Medical Schools that are right for you.

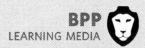

BPP LEARNING MEDIA

www.bpp.com/health

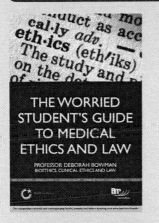

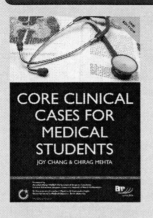

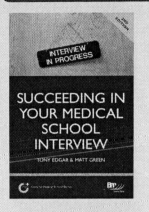

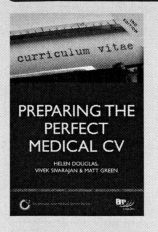